GW01464108

GLAZIERS & WINDOW BREAKERS

*The role of the
Secretary of State for Health,
in their own words*

A letter to the Secretary of State for Health

May 2015

Dear Secretary of State

Welcome to Richmond House. There is no handbook for the job you are doing and, by the almost unanimous testament of your predecessors, it will be the hardest job you have ever done.

However, what follows in this book is a history of the post and the wisdom of ten former incumbents – their experiences, their trials and what they learnt. Hopefully they will give you some insight into the challenges ahead to help prepare you. Their main messages are as follows:

- Regardless of where you have come from, the Department of Health is different. It has a different culture, different structures and different demands to any other department. From the unusual relationships at the top, with what used to be a trio of permanent secretaries – the NHS chief executive, permanent secretary and the chief medical officer – to the much more complex existing arrangements that involve a statutorily independent commissioning board along with a set of regulators and other arm's-length bodies.

- The NHS is also different to any other part of the public sector: it is at or near number one in the list of public priorities; much of the talent and knowledge about care is on the clinical front line, with the associated political power; and it carries out very high-risk activities. For these reasons, the NHS is never far from the headlines.

- There is an inescapable overlap between politics and the management of the NHS. Different boards, executives and laws have tried to give a structure to the relationship between the two, but one of the key challenges is recognising and deciding what is in the scope of the politicians and what is in the scope of the service. Different incumbents have taken wildly differing views as to the extent of the overlap, but there is overall consensus that politicians should not try to 'manage' the NHS.

- There are two major but intangible factors that influence this politics/management overlap:
  - Context will always influence the degree to which the secretary of state will see the need for intervention. Context could come in the form of an event such as a financial crisis in the NHS or a flu pandemic – or, as William Waldegrave puts it: 'The job of the Secretary of State for Health depends on whether you think the system, at any given time, is in need of policy reform.'

  - Your behaviour will tend to trump structures and legislation. When the scandal of quality of care at Mid Staffordshire NHS Foundation Trust came to light, both Alan Johnson and Andy Burnham overruled Monitor to do their job as they saw fit. Similarly, Jeremy Hunt has been appreciably more interventionist than was intended by the 2012 Health and Social Care Act introduced by his predecessor.

Finally, we would not presume to offer direct advice as to how you should do your job, but we did ask your predecessors for theirs.

Each was informed by their own tenure and, within this book, you can read their thoughts on a range of issues, from staff pay to service reform. But if one theme was dominant in their advice, it was – in the first few months of the job at least – to give yourself space to think.

'Buy time,' says Alan Milburn. 'The best political trick I ever pulled off was to publish a 10-year plan.' 'Have a good think,' says Frank Dobson. 'Which is out of fashion really isn't it, to sit down and have a good think?' 'Make no major speeches for at least a month,' recommends Alan Johnson. 'Find out exactly what's going on there.'

Fundamentally, you will have to decide how you want to approach the role – as Virginia Bottomley puts it, 'Sometimes you want a window breaker and sometimes you want a glazier. Ken was a window breaker and he was brilliant. But after that you get William Waldegrave who was a glazier… And then a new set of problems will arrive and you need a Ken to break the windows again.'

I hope you enjoy the book, which I think is a great read. Best wishes and good luck,

Dr Jennifer Dixon CBE
Chief Executive,
The Health Foundation

Acknowledgements

The Health Foundation and the authors are deeply indebted to the ten former Secretaries of State for Health who, at remarkably short notice, found time for the interviews featured in this book. We are also immensely grateful to Sir Alan Langlands and Brian Edwards who, at even shorter notice, read a late draft, correcting errors of fact and interpretation. Any remaining instances of either remain the authors' responsibility alone.

Contents

Part 1:

History & analysis

by Nicholas Timmins

Introduction

What is the role of the Secretary of State for Health? What should it be? How far, in an almost entirely tax-funded NHS, can health ministers be removed from the day-to-day operations of the NHS? How far should they be, if the service is to remain accountable to its patients, to taxpayers and to the public at large?

These are the core questions that lie behind this review. To put them another way, and in rather more detail, how far can the service be turned into a 'self-improving' one, to use Labour's phrase from the mid-2000s? One where ministers, and the health department, really do stand right back from operational matters and let the service itself – clinicians, managers and patients – drive improvement and change. How far can policy, which clearly lies in the purview of ministers, genuinely be separated from strategy, from operations and from management?

Will the demands of patients in their particular case, or indeed the demands of patients and the public collectively – expressed through their MPs and the media and on to the secretary of state in parliament – ensure that ultimately ministers cannot escape operational responsibility? Is that the inevitable – and quite correct – price to be paid, at least to some degree, in a tax-funded health system?

Or is it – even if the answer to that last question is 'yes' – possible to find a more constructive balance between ministerial responsibility and operational matters? And, if so, where does that balance lie?

To address these issues, ten former health secretaries kindly agreed to be interviewed about them, starting with the questions 'what is the role of the Secretary of State for Health? What should it be? And what was it when you were there?' The Health Foundation is immensely grateful to them for finding the time so to do.

This study, unsurprisingly, was prompted by the decision of Andrew Lansley, health secretary between May 2010 and September 2012, to create NHS England – a statutorily independent 'commissioning board' that has been dubbed 'the world's biggest quango' (an accolade that may not be entirely accurate, although it is certainly England's biggest).

Since April 2013 NHS England has been responsible for managing, in 2014/15 prices, some £97.5bn of the NHS's total £112bn budget in England – the money for the 'front line' so to speak, with the remainder going on public health, education and training, and assorted responsibilities that remain with the Department of Health itself.

This study does not seek to provide a definitive assessment of the success and/or failure of these new arrangements.

The arrangements are still immensely young – barely two-and-a-half years old. So far only one health secretary and two chief executives of NHS England have been in charge of them. So a final verdict on how well this has or has not worked will have to wait for another day.

But the very fact that an idea that has knocked around for decades has now become a reality – the creation of an arm's-length body, or a more BBC-like structure, or a governing board separate from ministers, or a Health Service Commission (the idea has taken many forms) – has provided a new focus for these questions.

These questions involve some long-standing tensions. Between localisation and centralisation – in terms of administration and management, but also in terms of how far there should be local or national political accountability. Between the interests of patients and those of taxpayers. And between the interests of the staff and those of the patients and their carers which, inevitably, are not always aligned. Tensions that have existed, not just since the formation of the NHS in 1948, but which were there – and which had to be resolved – in the run-up to its creation. In 1945 and in the run-up to the 1946 Act there were Cabinet battles over whether it should be a national health service, or one run by local government. The current proposals for 'Devo-Manc' in Manchester could yet see local government playing a much larger role.

Before we get to the health secretaries' views, however, it is important to note that each of them operated in an environment where the management of the NHS itself changed over the years. So – if readers can bear with it – a decent dose of history is required, even if it is a short and somewhat superficial one, and one which by no means covers all the changes to the NHS superstructure (the various tiers of authority and the various purchasing arrangements) over the years.

It is needed both to paint the backdrop of what each of the health secretaries inherited, and to dispel some myths.

A short history of health secretaries and the NHS

1948–1974
One of the biggest myths about the NHS is that it was deliberately set up in 1948 by Aneurin Bevan as a 'command and control' system to be run from Whitehall – or, more accurately from Jermyn Street where the department was then headquartered.

It is a myth that has been reinforced by almost every health secretary since at least the 1980s as, in various ways, they have sought to distinguish what they were up to from the bad old days of 'Soviet-style command and control' – to quote just one speech of Virginia Bottomley's in the 1990s.

It is a view reinforced by the famous Bevan quote that when a bedpan was dropped in Tredegar the sound would echo in the corridors of Whitehall – although I've never actually been able to find a reliable original source for this famous dictum, or the many variations of it that have been used.

It is a view reinforced by the almost equally famous 1937 observation of Douglas Jay that 'the gentlemen in Whitehall really do know best' – in fact, itself, a paraphrase. What he actually said was 'in the case of nutrition and health, just as in the case of education, the gentlemen in Whitehall really do know better what is good for the people than the people themselves'.

The Bevan aphorism is usually quoted as though it was something he profoundly desired; that he positively wanted the bedpans to echo in Whitehall. There is in fact a strong case that his words should be viewed the other way round. That what he was describing was something that he recognised to be an unwanted by-product of the system he had created. The case for this alternative view is there in what he said. And in what he did.

On 2 June 1948, a month before the launch of the NHS he made a speech to the Royal College of Nursing. According to the report in *Nursing Times*, he declared that after 5 July, there would be many complaints. The order paper of the House of Commons would be covered in questions. 'Every mistake which you make, I will bleed for,' he said. 'I shall be going about like St Sebastian, bleeding from a thousand javelins, so many people will be complaining.' They were complaining at the time, he said. But they weren't being heard. The arrival of the service would place 'a megaphone' in the hands of those who complained, although he predicted that the number would 'dwindle and dwindle… because *you* will be attending to them. All *I* shall be is a central receiver of complaints.'[1]

The italics there are my emphasis. But these hardly sound like the words of a man who saw the echoing of dropped bedpans to be something entirely desirable, or of someone who wanted to run the service by command and control. And certainly he did not set it up that way.

Hospitals were to be run by regional hospital boards, not from Whitehall and not as outposts of the Department of Health. The teaching hospitals retained an additional special status with their own boards of governors continuing to exist. It was Bevan himself who insisted that GPs should be independent contractors, not state or local government employees, and he did so in part because he wanted to ensure that patients had a choice of GP.

And when in 1950 Bevan appointed a senior civil servant, Sir Cyril Jones, to study the financial workings of the NHS as expenditure appeared to be running out of control, Bevan rejected Sir Cyril's recommendations. These included turning the regional hospital boards into purely planning bodies while the individual hospital management committees beneath them should become 'subject to direct control by the ministry' with civil servants posted out to them in order to ensure that.

Bevan's response was that 'there would have been no theoretical difficulty – there is none now – in having from the outset a tightly administered centralised service with all that would mean in the way of rigid uniformity, bureaucratic machinery and "red tape". But that was not the policy which we adopted when framing our legislation.

'While we are now – and rightly, I think – tightening up some of the elements of our financial control, we must remember that in framing the whole service we did deliberately come down in favour of maximum decentralisation to local bodies, a minimum of itemised central approval, and the exercise of financial control through global budgets.'[2]

As Rudolf Klein, the distinguished analyst of the NHS's history, has put it, the 1940s and 1950s were characterised 'by a philosophy of administration which saw policy as the product of interaction rather than as the imposition of national plans'.

'The centre provided the financial framework and advice about desirable objectives. It left the periphery free to work out the details… The centre, quite simply, did not know best – and indeed could not know best.' Even when it had a clear view about what was desirable 'it did not perceive itself to be in a position to command. It could educate, it could inspire, it could stimulate. To have done more would have run counter to the values of localism… and challenged the right of [clinical] professionals to decide on the content of their work.' It was,

Klein says, a case of 'policy making through exhortation'. As one civil servant put it in evidence to a parliamentary committee 'the minister seeks always to act by moral suasion'.[2]

The NHS was, of course, a national organisation in that it had, and still largely has, national terms and conditions. The department issued many circulars on that and on many other matters, including broader policy aims. Roughly one every three days throughout the 1950s. But how far the thousands – literally in those days thousands – of individual hospitals acted on them was a matter for them and for the regional hospital boards which retained a distinct, decidedly local, independence from the centre. And that remained pretty much the case through the 1960s.

Even Enoch Powell's mighty 1962 Hospital Plan, which promised 90 new hospitals and the remodelling, on various degrees of scale, of some 490 more, became, in Rudolf Klein's words, a 'negotiated order'. Not only that, but, as it turned out, a much delayed one. As civil servants told a parliamentary inquiry, the department could 'advise' the regional hospital boards, it could 'discuss' the plan and seek to 'persuade', but it would not dictate. Not least because 'it is not easy for us centrally… to form a judgement of the precise needs of each regional board'.[2] The same applied to Powell's other great initiative, the 'setting of the torch to the funeral pyre' of the great Victorian lunatic asylums, announced in his famous 'water towers' speech.[*] It was to take 30 years for the last of them to close.

Indeed at the end of the 1960s, Richard Crossman, Labour's health secretary (strictly speaking the first Secretary of State for Social Services), described the relationship with the service as follows: 'You don't have in the regional hospital boards

---

[*]   In this speech, Powell spoke about the huge psychiatric institutions, saying:
    'There they stand, isolated, majestic, imperious, brooded over by the gigantic water-tower and chimney combined, rising unmistakable and daunting out of the countryside––the asylums which our forefathers built with such immense solidity.' These, he said, were 'the defences we have to storm' setting 'the torch to [their] funeral pyre.'

a number of obedient civil servants carrying out central orders… You have a number of powerful, semi-autonomous boards whose relation to me was much more like the relations of a Persian satrap to a weak Persian emperor. If the emperor tried to enforce his authority too far he lost his throne, or at least lost his resources, or something broke down.'

The department was perfectly capable of putting out detailed circulars on precise requirements for building specifications which were expected to be followed. So the distinction should not be pushed too far. But, certainly up to the mid-1970s, and on most measures until the mid-1980s, the NHS was essentially an *administered* service rather than a *managed* one. One where policy, in so far as it could be enforced, was enforced by persuasion, discussion and advice. Not by central planning, and most certainly not by command and control.

One should not underestimate the power of a phone call from one of the department's senior civil servants. But health ministers up to the 1980s and indeed beyond, and doubtless even today, would say that in practice there was damn all command available, and, for much of the time, more or less bugger all control.

1974–1983

This, in time, led to frustration. Ministers were indeed accountable for the NHS and had to answer many gruesomely detailed questions about it in parliament. But the sense steadily grew, not just in the ministry but in the Treasury and elsewhere, that there were too few levers that could be pulled at the centre with any sense of certainty that anything would change on the ground. For example, by the 1970s there had been, for many years, a developing policy for 'care in the community', not least for the mentally ill, people with learning difficulties, as well as for others in the so-called 'Cinderella services'. Progress, while real, was snail-like. Ministers could exhort. They could not execute.

The mighty 1974 reorganisation of the NHS was in part an answer to that. It was also many others things – not least an attempt (which partially failed) to unify the service.

Bevan's original dispensation had left much with local government – for example district nursing and health visiting, midwifery, the ambulance and the schools service, along with public health, with the best (though not the worst) of the local authority medical officers of health being powerful and effective figures. 1974 brought all of this together. Health authorities replaced purely hospital boards, acquiring a broader population remit. The reorganisation, however, failed also to unify what we would now call social care with health. Social care remained with the councils. Nor did the reorganisation bring GPs under more direct management, although both ideas were extensively trailed and debated.

The mid-1970s was, of course, the apogee of faith in planning in the UK. The near absolute belief that the state could plan and run services better, and, indeed could do so in parts of the private as well as the public sector. This vision was held by both the main political parties at the time, even if to varying degrees. It was a faith that was to fall, rapidly and spectacularly, out of favour, at least among the Conservatives.

So the 1974 reorganisation, the product of Sir Keith Joseph as the social services secretary, did indeed introduce a planning system into the NHS for the first time, even if it proved initially to be highly tortuous, and eventually rather weak.

It was introduced with two slogans. The first was 'maximum delegation downwards, but maximum accountability upwards' – the very phrase capturing the tension between localism and centralism. The second was 'consensus management'. This saw finance officers and senior clinical staff – chiefly, but not exclusively, doctors and nurses – brought onto health authority boards and onto district management teams as nominally equal partners to sit alongside administrators. And, at this stage, hospital and health authority managers were still very much administrators, if often powerful ones, and were named as such.

In administrative terms, this was part of the weakening of the autonomy of the medical profession. One of the first major dilutions of the unwritten compact at the beginning of the NHS. Namely, that the taxpayer would fund the NHS but the medical professionals would largely be trusted, individually as well as collectively, to decide what should be provided. The retreat of the profession's ability to influence policy over how the NHS was run is a huge subject in its own right, though one that is largely, but not entirely, outside the scope of this study.

In so far as there is any truth in the NHS having ever been in practice a 'command and control' system, the 1974 reorganisation was an attempt to introduce at least an element of both. The search for a set of policy levers that would indeed give ministers, as representatives of the taxpayer, more power to implement the policies they set out. An ability to plan, linked to a mechanism to deliver.

In the words of Sir Patrick Nairne, the permanent secretary who inherited the results of this mighty reorganisation, 1974 became a case of 'tears about tiers'. The new structure of regional, area and district health authorities proved mightily bureaucratic. The teaching hospitals lost their independent boards of governors and were placed under the area health authorities – a melancholy little plaque in the boardroom at Guy's recording the final meeting of its governors in their 248th year. That plaque, a dozen years later, was to catch the eye of a Downing Street adviser, leading first to the creation of NHS trusts and, many more years on, to their offspring: NHS foundation trusts.[3]

If 1974 saw the NHS become much more bureaucratic and, to a very limited degree, more of a command and control system, it also became much more politicised through the introduction of local authority members on to the boards of health authorities.

Councillors had indeed been on regional hospital boards. But they had been there as individuals, not as nominees or formal representatives. The reorganisation coincided with a tough time for the economy, and thus health spending. And an additional voice had been added to the formal mechanisms of the NHS in the shape of community health councils (CHCs) who were there, for the first time, to represent patients. As the money tightened, however, both the councillors and the CHCs voted themselves the role of critics – a stance that was enhanced by the tendency of medical and nursing members of the authorities to act as though they were representatives of their professions, rather than what they were formally appointed to be – informed individuals. As the unions and governments of both colour clashed repeatedly in the 1970s over pay and much else, the net result was that the level of political debate about the NHS escalated, with many on the health authorities publicly blaming any and every problem on a lack of resources from central government rather than anything else.

Enoch Powell – who, in my view, despite the 'rivers of blood', must rate as one of the half-dozen great health ministers – once observed of a tax-funded NHS that it endowed 'everyone providing as well as using it with a vested interest in denigrating it' – in the hope that the result would be more money. The 1974 reorganisation handed them all a bullhorn. Thus the level of accountability demanded from health ministers – if not necessarily their sense of what they could practically be held accountable for – rose.[3]

Initially the reorganisation did little to make administrators feel they were any more directly accountable to the ministry than in the past. It is at this time your author started reporting on the NHS, and back then many administrators saw themselves as public guardians of the NHS locally – frequently speaking out individually and publicly against assorted bits of government policy, with little sense that they feared dismissal from above; something that is seen somewhat less often these days, save where they are speaking on behalf of at least some sort of NHS collective body.

Glacially, however, that began to change. In 1975 the department added to the planning system a programme budget. That allowed it to work out broadly where the NHS was spending its cash – showing for example that a falling birth rate had not been matched by a reduction in maternity services, thus allowing money to be diverted from that to community care for the geriatric and mentally ill, and for growth in acute services to be restrained to achieve the same thing. Broad targets for changed priorities could now not only be set, but monitored.

Equally, again slowly but again surely, the regional chairs of the health authorities became increasingly powerful figures. In time, as we shall see, some became despotic. These were people who, when they took on board what the minister wanted, began to demand action from their own regional administrators and staff, and so on down the line. How far that applied varied distinctly across the country. But all this – a planning system – did indeed begin to introduce a little more command and a little more control, and somewhat less freedom for administration locally to decide whether or not to comply with the wishes of the centre.

Further evidence that it is a myth that the NHS was created as a 'command and control' system comes in the voluminous report of the Royal Commission on the NHS in 1979. It reviewed the 1974 reorganisation. But nowhere does it contain the phrase 'command and control'. It does reflect the many bitter complaints about the bureaucracy created by the new tiers and matching advisory machinery.[4] But one of its key observations is that 'in principle health ministers… are expected to have detailed knowledge of and influence over the NHS. In practice, however, this is neither possible nor desirable and detailed ministerial accountability for the NHS is largely a constitutional fiction. That is not to say that it is without virtues'. It quoted approvingly a memorandum from the department that its 'oversight of, and assistance to authorities is generally more by administrative guidance than by legislation'.

The full scale of the bureaucracy of the 1974 reorganisation was unpacked by Patrick Jenkin [Baron Jenkin of Roding] in the 1982 reorganisation. Area health authorities were abolished and there was a marked reduction of some of the highly convoluted advisory machinery that had accompanied the 1974 restructure.

'Consensus management', however, remained. At its best it worked well. But the demand for 'consensus' on local decisions meant that anyone and everyone from the doctor to the nurse to the finance officer to the administrator had, at least potentially, a veto. Too often the result was lowest common denominator decisions on any change that was proposed, not highest common factor ones, and sometimes no decision at all. As Norman Fowler, Secretary of State for Social Services between 1981 and 1987, has put it, 'consensus management was basically a way of avoiding decisions'.[5]

Jenkin recalls of his time between 1979 and 1981 'you issued circulars and you didn't know what the effect was going to be'. But he had meetings 'from time to time' with the regional chairmen and they were 'the levers I could pull to make sure something happened'.[5]

It is now that we enter the territory of the health secretaries interviewed here.

The 1980s

Ken Clarke arrived as a health minister – not yet secretary of state – in 1982 when proper cash limits for the NHS were biting for the first time. There was little real terms growth after NHS pay and price rises had been allowed for. The public discourse was dominated by 'cuts'. And the longest industrial dispute in 50 years, and the NHS's longest ever, was just kicking off.

'The problem is that there wasn't a management system worth the name,' Clarke says. 'There was next to no management information of any kind, no one knew what the devil we were spending the money on, and the whole thing was dominated by political campaigning. It wasn't command and control… though I was supposed to command and control.'

To get any growth in services, costs had to be constrained without damaging the service itself. The result was a vast plethora of initiatives that included some rather arbitrary manpower targets – instituted because staff numbers were exploding and some authorities were literally unable to state how many people they employed. There was pressure to sell off nurses' homes, to rationalise job advertising and much else, plus a hotly contested requirement to put cleaning, catering and laundry out to competitive tender. 'So I did do some command and control,' Clarke says, although history shows that administrators and health authority members became increasingly resentful of these centrally dictated efficiency drives.

Clarke and Norman Fowler, as his boss, also ramped up the influence of the politically appointed health authority chairs, at both regional and district level. They refused to reappoint those who refused to deliver on the compulsory competitive tendering of support services, or who sided in public with the staff in the nine-month pay dispute. Refusing to reappoint them was 'the only lever I had, and the one I continued to pull all the time,' Clarke says. 'I gradually got rid of the ones [the chairs] who used to go on strike with the staff and stand on the picket lines, and got in people who were good, local businessmen – not very political, most of them. That was regarded as a real novelty. I used to describe them as my "health cabinet".'

He and Fowler, with the chairs, also instituted formal annual reviews of each of the 14 regions. Reviews of their performance against agreed targets, and therefore reviews of the performance of the regional administrators, which were then replicated down the line to each region's districts – but not to the units that were directly responsible for the management of hospitals. This was the very beginnings of performance management in the NHS.

One aspect of the relationship of ministers to the service is neatly captured in one of Clarke's stories. 'One of my first introductions to the service was that I had to go to close a maternity hospital in Clement Freud's constituency [the Isle of Ely]… A great demonstration took place, and they were moving the babies inside to try to give me the impression there were more than there were. I met the local grand consultants, the obstetricians, who told me ferociously – addressing a minister of state in an absolutely James Robertson Justice way – that I had got to close this place. And they had all agreed that they were not going to accept any more referrals to it. "It was dangerous!" – and they had a better facility in some local East Anglian town.'

'So I said: "Come out with me and say that to all these women and these television cameras outside who are waving babies at me." And they refused. Absolutely refused. And it turned out they had not shared this opinion with anybody but me and the doctors from whom they were refusing to accept referrals. One of them said, "That is your job, we are not prepared to do that." That is a silly story, but it is a true story. It was my first introduction to the fact that some of the medical profession had no time at all for those who did manage the service, but were not prepared to accept the slightest responsibility for managing any change.

'In fact I closed more hospitals than most people had hot dinners – old Victorian workhouses which were called "geriatric hospitals" but which suddenly became centres of clinical excellence when their closure was proposed.'

If Clarke and Fowler were worried about the management of the service, so was Margaret Thatcher, the prime minister. Largely at her instigation, Roy Griffiths, the managing director of Sainsbury's – at the time by far the most successful supermarket in Britain – was brought in, initially to do an inquiry into manpower that soon became one into the management of the NHS. Clarke bristled. 'There I was clattering about, contracting out this and manpowering that in an attempt to get some management into the service, and here's this bloke they want to bring in to spend 12 months doing a study… in fact Roy produced a very good report. My reluctance about it turned out to be a terrible mistake.'[*]

In the entire history of the NHS, in my view the Griffiths report is one of its three most important documents – alongside the Guillebaud report of 1956[6] which rescued the service financially and Ken Clarke's later white paper *Working for Patients*[7] which introduced the purchaser/provider split with which we still live. The Griffiths report was easily the most idiosyncratic of the three.

Griffiths produced a mere 14-page 'letter' in February 1983, not a formal report. It was, so to speak, written backwards. It began with seven pages of recommendations, followed by seven of diagnosis, while being entirely shorn of the formal evidence beloved of official inquiries.[8]

Its essential message was encapsulated in one ringing phrase. That 'if Florence Nightingale were carrying her lamp through the corridors of the NHS today, she would almost certainly be searching for the people in charge'.

The recommendation from Griffiths and his team of three other business people was, in essence, that 'consensus management' with its 'lowest common denominator decisions' should go. General managers – regardless of discipline – should be appointed at every level of the NHS. The review process – the setting of budgets and objectives and the monitoring of performance and outputs in so far as they were

[*] For accounts of the origins, nature and impact of the Griffiths report see: Brian Edwards and Margaret Fall. *The executive years of the NHS*. Nuffield Trust. Radcliffe Publishing, 2005; Nicholas Timmins. *The five giants: A biography of the Welfare State*. HarperCollins, 2001; Rudolf Klein. *The new politics of the NHS*. Any edition but in the 7th Edition pp117–123.

measurable – that Fowler and Clarke had instituted should be strengthened, and extended down to the hospital level. Doctors should not just be eligible to be general managers. They should take responsibility for their own budgets at hospital level because 'their decisions largely dictate the use of all resources, and they must accept the management responsibility which goes with clinical freedom'. And the centre should be revamped.

'A small, strong general management body is necessary at the centre (and that is almost all that is necessary at the centre for the management of the NHS).' This NHS Management Board, with its chair acting as a general manager or chief executive for the NHS, should be answerable to an NHS Supervisory Board, chaired by the secretary of state, with the permanent secretary, the chief medical officer, and the management board chair on it, along with two or three non-executives.

And it really was, in many ways, that simple. The goal was genuine devolution of responsibility down the line 'to the point where action can effectively be taken', with accountability going back up it. An attempt, in a sense, to make a reality of the slogan that had accompanied the 1974 reorganisation. The department, the inquiry said, should 'rigorously prune many of its existing activities… the centre is still too much involved in too many of the wrong things and too little involved in some that really matter… units and authorities are being swamped with directives, without being given direction'.

The word 'command' does not appear anywhere in the Griffiths report. But 'control' does. Repeatedly. 'By general management,' it says, 'we mean the responsibility drawn together in one person, at different levels of the organisation, for planning, implementation and control of performance'.

Put another way, here was a mechanism that provided more of a lever for ministers to set policy and for something down the line to happen as a result – another turn of the performance management screw – even if the primary objective remained to get decisions taken at the point 'where action can effectively be taken'. As a result, even within the Griffiths solution, the tension between centralism and localism that had been at the heart of the NHS since its foundation still played out.

This was, however, undoubtedly the moment when the NHS moved from being largely an *administered* system to more of a *managed* one.

A powerful case can be made that the Griffiths report saved the NHS – by putting someone in charge. Certainly without the arrival of general management there would have been no one to implement *Working for Patients* with its creation of allegedly self-governing NHS trusts and the introduction of the purchaser/provider split some eight years later.

Less noticed at the time – and less analysed since – was that the report also reinforced the role of the politically appointed chairs at both regional and district level. It was they who were to appoint the general managers. And they retained a separate reporting line – separate from that of the managers – to the very ministers who had appointed them. Over time, and particularly after the 1991 reforms, their influence was to grow.

The recommendations were profoundly controversial. The Royal College of Nursing launched a huge advertising campaign asking why the NHS nurses should be run by someone 'who doesn't know their coccyx from their humerus'. Fowler agonised for eight months over accepting the report. The implementation circular went through 14 drafts before being issued – in part because while many of the civil servants in the department liked the report's recommendations for strong local management, they strongly disliked the threat to their empire posed by a small, strong and separate local management board. In the end, Fowler bit the bullet. Both the management board and the supervisory board came into existence, more or less as Griffiths had recommended.

The other key element of the Griffiths report was that it was the first formal attempt to distance politicians from the day-to-day management of the service – through its mainland Europe-like, company-like, structure of a supervisory and management board. The secretary of state was to chair the supervisory board, not the management one. The role of the supervisory board was to be 'oversight' of the NHS. Setting objectives, approving the budget, taking strategic decisions, receiving reports on performance – not managing the service. That, in theory, was for the management board. Very deliberately, these changes were designed to take effect with no requirement for legislation. They were new management arrangements, not – as in the case of the 2012 Act – new statutory ones.

The subsequent history of the management board is long and tortuous. It went through assorted incarnations of being a board, and then a management executive, then an executive, each of which was recast in various ways at various times. It is well set out in *The executive years of the NHS by* Brian Edwards and Margaret Fall.[9]

Only the most crucial changes will be outlined here, the interest of this study being more in the relation of ministers to the service, and thus what happened to the political 'distancing' arrangement of the supervisory board.

The short answer is that the board fell into desuetude. It met for the first time in October 1983, and regularly for the first two years of its life. It met less frequently thereafter. In the run up to the 1987 general election, its meetings were repeatedly cancelled, and when Fowler and Clarke moved on in the wake of the general election, John Moore, Fowler's successor, had little understanding of it and little interest in it. The board had helped oversee the introduction of general management, although its impact is hard to assess, not least because it met in private (as did the management board) and neither body published any minutes. It is clear, however, that its *precise* role rapidly became decidedly *imprecise* as ministers in practice remained in charge and still took most of the crucial decisions. As Norman Fowler put it, in a phrase that in part became the title of his political memoir: 'Officials advise. Ministers decide.' And that applied equally to the supervisory board. Indeed, as early as November 1986 the arrangements had been rejigged so that, while the supervisory board continued, Tony Newton, the health minister, started to chair the management board, an arrangement that clearly diluted the theoretical split between the two. The supervisory board was finally scrapped in June 1988. It had met only six times over the previous two years. Len Peach, the chief executive of the management board at the time judged that it had become 'a waste of time… ministers got bored with it… they had already heard the debates beforehand'.[9]

By now the NHS was deep into the huge financial crisis of 1987 that led first to Margaret Thatcher's review of the NHS, then the return of Ken Clarke, this time as health secretary. The NHS was well on the way to the monumental row that accompanied *Working for Patients* with its introduction of the purchaser/provider split, 'self-governing' NHS trusts and GP fundholding.* The so-called NHS 'internal market'.

As the white paper was launched in early 1989, the NHS Management Board was reorganised once again. It became the NHS Management Executive with Duncan Nichol as its chief executive.

Nichol was clear – there is an official circular to this effect – that 'separating the role of managers from ministers will be a prime consideration. The implementation of policy will be the responsibility of the management executive'.[9] And with the huge undertaking of introducing the purchaser/provider split under way, Clarke reintroduced the strategic/management split at the centre. He created an NHS Policy Board to sit above

---

* For an account of the origins of the review and its immediate impact see :Timmins N. *The five giants: A biography of the Welfare State*. HarperCollins, 2001; Klein R. *The New Politics of the NHS*.Radcliffe, 2006. For more academic assessments of the longer-term impact of the reforms see: Klein R. *The new politics of the NHS* ; Le Grand J et al (eds) *Learning from the NHS internal market: a review of the evidence*. The King's Fund, 1998.

the management executive, its membership consisting of a mix of ministers, senior officials, three business people and a couple of the regional chairs.[9]

Its intention was at least as much to provide some strategic oversight to the massive changes in the way the NHS was to function as it was to distance ministers from management – although Clarke did seek to signal that was indeed the intention by insisting that the headquarters of the management executive be in Leeds, not in Whitehall or London. It was a decision that, over time, exhausted many of the most senior people on the management executive as they spent countless hours on trains up and down to London, endlessly dragging behind them an overnight suitcase.

Of the early meetings of the board, one civil servant recalls that they consisted 'of the secretary of state [Clarke] dominating the meeting, both by his manner – he smoked a large cigar in a no smoking area – and by the way he used the opportunity to expound his own views, opening up certain areas for discussion while keeping others tight'.[9]

The 1990s

William Waldegrave took over from Clarke as Secretary of State for Health barely five months before the purchaser/provider split went live in April 1991. He refreshed the membership of the policy board.

Waldegrave's judgement is that the policy board 'did some good in its early days' – in overseeing the establishment of the purchaser/provider split and the resulting structures. But his overall judgement is that 'it didn't do all that much' because the policy board/management executive split repeatedly came back to 'the inherent difficulty of the whole thing – is it possible, in any business or in any organisation, truly to separate policy from execution?' This is an issue to which we will return, while simply noting for now that Stephen Dorrell scrapped the policy board in 1995.

The 1991 reforms – the purchaser/provider split – came, as do almost all government reforms, not just in health, with its paradoxes. Its rhetoric was that it was about decentralisation. The substitution of some market-like mechanisms for direct management of the service from the centre (in so far as there was in fact any direct management). By implication, that meant less day-to-day involvement of ministers in running it. So self-governing NHS hospitals were to compete for the business of two sets of purchasers – health authorities and GP fundholders.

Paradoxically, however, the purchaser/provider split also strengthened the control of the centre. For a start, a huge wealth of guidance and rules poured out of it as everyone tried to work out how to make this so-called 'internal market' work, without it causing total disruption.

In addition, the arrival of allegedly self-governing NHS trusts saw the creation of many more boards, and thus many more, decidedly hands-on, chairs. Many of them were business people and Conservative party supporters. All of them were committed to making the internal market work. Waldegrave and his successor Virginia Bottomley may have been much more emollient figures than Ken Clarke. But the net result was something of a reign of terror as the new activist chairmen (and they mainly were men) along with the hospital general managers – who had all, unilaterally and overnight, restyled themselves 'chief executives' – alighted on poorer performers with the instruction to 'clear your desk by tomorrow'. The culture became so poisonous that in June 1992 Duncan Nichol had to appeal publicly for an end to such 'macho management'.[3]

Griffiths and the new purchaser/provider split had thus between them produced a dual reporting line: a managerial one through the management executive, while at the same time enhancing the separate, politically appointed one – at the very least an 'eyes and ears' line – from chairs to ministers.

Both made it possible for ministers to institute top-down reform – issuing instructions about priorities and having some hope that they would be implemented. It was a possibility that ministers and the department could not resist to the point where Alan Langlands, Nichol's successor, promised in 1994 to try to reduce the flood of paper pouring out into the service. As he put it, 'when you have more than fifty priorities, the truth is that you have no priorities at all.'[10] By now, the tendency of NHS management, to borrow the phrase popularised a decade later by David Nicholson and Patricia Hewitt, to 'look up, not look out' was becoming increasingly established, when the price of perceived failure could too often be your job.

This reign of terror gradually eased and the power of chairs slowly diluted. The introduction of at least nominally 'self-governing' NHS trusts, with district health authorities and GP fundholders doing the purchasing from them, inevitably called into question the role of regional health authorities. These were subject to repeated restructuring, culminating in their abolition in 1996. The 14 regions were scrapped and replaced by eight regional offices of the NHS management executive – and later on by four – with their officials becoming civil servants. Virginia Bottomley presented all this, when it was announced in 1993, as 'a lighter approach geared to developing the potential of purchasing.' And there was truth in that. But, as she said in her statement, the management executive also took on 'a clearer identity as the headquarters of the national health service.'[11] Or as Alan Langlands was later to put it, the NHS now had for the first time, through the management executive and its regional offices, 'a single, corporate, management structure at the centre of the NHS.'[3]

The regional chairs – who no longer had authorities to chair – in fact survived because Bottomley still valued them as her 'Lord Lieutenants'. The eyes and ears who would tell her 'what she did not want to hear.'[9] But their role was much reduced, becoming in time essentially one of advising on appointments, including to the boards of NHS trusts, in their patch. An NHS Appointments Commission was later to further depoliticise these appointments while also, along the way, doing something about the gender balance, if not much about the ethnic mix. The dual reporting line gradually diluted and then, in Labour's time, disappeared.

One further, rarely discussed, factor increased the centralising tendency. It may sound slightly technical, but it matters. The permanent secretary of the department had always been its accounting officer – personally answerable to parliament, chiefly through the Public Accounts Committee, for the safeguarding of public funds and ensuring that money is only spent as parliament intended. The NHS chief executive, however, and in time chief executives further down the NHS food chain also became accountable officers, *personally* responsible not only for that but, as the appointment letter says, 'day-to-day operations.' The Treasury's accounting officer letter is often said by new chief executives at all levels in the NHS to be the most terrifying thing they receive on appointment. During Alan Langlands' six and a half year tenure as NHS chief executive, for example, he faced no fewer than 28 hearings in front of the Public Accounts Committee – and its hearings, as anyone who has ever attended them can testify, can become a form of blood sport. When personally answerable for NHS performance it is hardly surprising that successive NHS chief executives felt the need for some degree of influence and control.

Thus, while a key aim of the so-called 'internal market' was to push purchasing and operational decisions down the line to the point where they could most effectively be taken, the new arrangements in the mid-1990s can also be seen, as Rudolf Klein has put it, though in slightly different words, as a new high for the tide of centralisation that had been slowly creeping up the beach.[2]

Furthermore, thanks to a separate but related review in 1994,[12] the management executive also gained a significant role in policy formation and thus in advice to ministers on matters other than implementation. The department's policy division was largely broken up. The idea was that policy had to pay regard to the realities of implementation and to its costs.[9] In its earliest incarnation, this shift of policy advice towards that of experienced NHS managers worked well. It was to work much less happily later.

The 2000s

Over the following years, slowly but surely, the power of the management executive vis-à-vis the power of the civil servants in the Department of Health rose, to the point where – as Scott Greer and Holly Jarman have put it in their study of the department – it became 'a department dominated by the NHS' or more precisely by NHS managers.[13] This trend – the gradual disempowerment of the department's traditional civil servants – was reinforced when Labour arrived in 1997 and it became special advisers, both within the department and at Number 10, rather than civil servants, who became the key policy advisers (and deciders) for ministers.

With Tony Blair's promise effectively to double NHS spending in real terms, and along with the NHS Plan in 2000, came the myriad waiting time targets – an absolutely command and control approach to that issue. Among hospital chief executives, the waiting time goals became known as 'P45 targets', as Blair and his delivery unit held monthly stocktakes with health ministers to ensure that progress continued. The department now had some decidedly well-oiled machinery that was capable of ringing hospital chief executives weekly where insufficient progress was being made.

As Alan Milburn has put it – and this continued well beyond his time until the targets were reached – 'it was relentless focus. The prime minister holding me to account, the delivery unit holding the department to account, me holding the department to account and the department holding chief executives to account – with the NHS knowing that this was the absolute top priority, because people were suffering and dying.'

Or as Duncan Selbie, a former NHS manager who was the director general of performance and programmes in the department at the time, has put it, 'No one ever got fired if they were trying hard, and any amount of effort went in to help. But for the first time in the NHS there was a clear line of sight from the prime minister down to the chief executives on the front line, and again, for the first time, there were consequences.'* The fact that it was clinicians, and not just managers, who made the changes needed was not entirely lost to sight. But it was the chief executives who were held accountable.

The disempowerment of the traditional civil service reached its peak in 2000. Following the departure of Alan Langlands as NHS chief executive, Alan Milburn, the health secretary, took the remarkable decision to merge the jobs of permanent secretary and chief executive of the NHS.

As Greer and Jarman have calculated, by 2005, when Nigel Crisp departed and this unhappy experiment of the two jobs becoming one ended, of the top 30 leadership positions in the department, only one was held by a classic civil servant – the others being NHS managers, clinical 'czars' or recruits from the wider public and private sectors.[13] It is possible to take issue with those precise figures; but the essential point is well made.

Unfortunately, this generation of managers proved in the longer run to be good at neither policy nor some crucial aspects of management. Quite remarkably, the service plunged into a significant overspend despite record levels of growth.

---

* For a detailed account of how waiting times were driven down, see Road To Recovery. *Financial Times* weekend magazine, March 13/14, 2010 pp14–29.

Ministers struggled to find the advice that would help them bring full coherence to the mixture of choice, competition and foundation trust status, plus wider use of the private sector, that had become the key drivers of NHS policy. This approach was intended to produce a 'self-improving' NHS and reduce the reliance on 'targets and terror' (in other words, command and control) as the means of raising the quality and quantity of services.* Under Patricia Hewitt in 2005, the jobs of the permanent secretary and the NHS chief executive were once again separated, and the traditional civil service started to come back into its own.

Labour's time also, however, saw three key – and on the whole successful – distancing mechanisms. The first was the arrival in 1999 of NICE, now the National Institute for Health and Care Excellence. NICE has not taken all the heat out of the decisions about which treatments the NHS should and should not provide. But with one or two exceptions – Patricia Hewitt urging primary care trusts to provide Herceptin ahead of NICE's appraisal and the ongoing issues around the Cancer Drugs Fund – NICE has shielded ministers from having to make these key decisions. Mainly because they have allowed it to. There is no statutory requirement for ministers to accept NICE's decisions.

The second is the Independent Reconfiguration Panel, set up by John Reid but initially used by Patricia Hewitt and Alan Johnson. Reconfigurations are referred to it. It provides a stamp of approval or otherwise, sometimes with some amendment to the original proposition, and makes recommendations to ministers. In other words, it provides an element of independent and clinical judgement to local NHS proposals for change. Ministers can shelter behind its verdict, removing them from the management decision. As Alan Johnson put it, 'I didn't entirely tie my hands' by saying he

---

* The fine phrase 'targets and terror' was coined by Gwyn Bevan of the London School of Economics.

would never overturn its recommendations. But he did tell parliament 'I can foresee no circumstances in which I would intervene.'

The third was the Co-operation and Competition Panel which Johnson set up to hear complaints about the breach of procurement and competition law as Labour's policy of competition and choice to produce this 'self-improving' NHS moved to the fore and that law came into play.* The panel was purely advisory, not statutory. Ministers could have rejected its advice. But again, quietly and effectively, and because ministers allowed it to, it took difficult management and indeed legal decisions – on whether to intervene – out of the hands of ministers. It left those who had a complaint with the choice of accepting its verdict or going to court. It never got taken to court.

Aside from these three specific mechanisms, of course, the whole thrust of Labour's reforms was intended to take politicians out of direct management. Foundation trusts were statutory bodies, set up as public benefit corporations part-way between the public and private sectors – in an attempt to make the freedoms that NHS trusts had theoretically enjoyed, but had gradually lost, a permanent reality. They were overseen by their own regulator, Monitor, which was the only body which could approve them, and technically it was only Monitor, not ministers, that could fire their boards and chief executives when performance went awry. The Care Quality Commission (CQC) had become a full-blown NHS inspectorate, with its own ability, technically without ministerial approval, to be able to close hospitals. The purchaser/provider split, with its mimicking of market-like mechanisms, rather than those of direct management, survived.

---

* For an account of how procurement and competition law came into the NHS see: Timmins N. *Never again: The story of the Health and Social Care Act 2012.* Institute for Government and the King's Fund, 2012.

The 2010s

It is against this background that Andrew Lansley legislated in 2012, making the mistake, in some people's eyes at least, of writing it all down in law.

The Health and Social Care Act is recent enough – and large enough – not to have to go through all its measures.[*] Key to it was Lansley's view that the way the NHS was to be managed and operated had to be written down in tablets of legislative stone so that it became 'permanent'.

'The evidence of the past was very clear,' he has said. 'That because the nature of the legislation was that you change the secretary of state and you can change the policy on virtually everything in the NHS, because the health service at any given time was basically what the secretary of state under the legislation decided it would be.'

His white paper was littered with phrases about ending 'political micro-management', 'political control' and 'political meddling'. Both his new commissioning board and the providers were to be freed from 'day-to-day political interference'.[14] His goal, he said, was to allow the NHS 'to take a more autonomous long-term view of their own role… [knowing] that things would not change just at the behest of the secretary of state, or even more a change of government.' Thus it would no longer be possible, for example, for Labour's policy to change from the active promotion of choice and competition under the Blairites to Andy Burnham's declaration as secretary of state in 2009 that the NHS was to be its own 'preferred provider'.

To borrow a phrase of Nigel Edwards at the time,[15] perhaps the most important thing to understand about Lansley's reform is that it made the NHS less of an organisation and more of an eco-system.

The NHS was no longer to be an organisation with a chief executive at its centre, however little power that chief

---

[*] For an account of the Act and its passage see: Timmins N. *Never again: The story of the Health and Social Care Act 2012.* Institute for Government and the King's Fund, 2012.

executive had in reality to engineer real change at the local level. It became instead more of an eco-system – something much closer to a regulated industry that operated without a single management chain. NHS England was no longer the headquarters of the NHS. It was instead merely a commissioner and an overseer of commissioners, even if it was a powerful one through which almost all the money flowed. It could not, however, even set NHS prices (the tariff) on its own. That task was to be shared with Monitor. But Monitor – in addition to retaining its statutory oversight of foundation trusts – also acquired a statutory responsibility for enforcing procurement and competition law, operating beneath the Competition and Markets Authority. The Trust Development Authority (TDA) became responsible for those organisations not yet ready to become foundation trusts – and for those which would never get there. Clinical commissioning groups did the bulk of local purchasing, with the boundaries between that and specialist commissioning already starting to move over time. In addition to Monitor and the TDA's regulation (though the TDA strictly speaking is not a regulator) there was the CQC which could place its own requirements on NHS organisations to improve. Between them and the host of other bodies that came to litter the NHS landscape – Public Health England, Health Education England, clinical senates, academic health science centres and networks, strategic clinical networks, and so on – all this was meant to provide a series of incentives and penalties, duties and pressures that would produce the 'self-improving' NHS of Labour's dreams. One where ministers merely set the priorities and the outcomes desired through a rolling annual mandate, and then left the NHS alone to deliver it. Or as one of David Cameron's special advisers was later, somewhat cynically and despairingly to put it, what was devised was, at least in theory, 'a perfectly incentivised perpetual motion machine'.[16]

As David Cameron and his colleagues were soon to discover, thanks to Lansley, ministers really had foregone command and control in the NHS – on paper at least. Although, as we shall see from the interviews, that did not stop them, regardless of the legislation, from seeking to reinstate at least a degree of control.

Lansley's declared aim of creating an NHS 'free from day-to-day political interference', was something that many had yearned for over the years – that yearning perhaps being an example of 'be careful for what it is you wish'.

The idea of an independent NHS board – or some version of it – has roots that stretch way back into history, although the precise definition of what sort of board should run the NHS was often missing, and, when it was present, varied over the years. The British Medical Association trailed the idea in 1970. The 1979 Royal Commission reported that 'the establishment of an independent health commission or board to manage the NHS was one of the solutions most frequently advocated in evidence. There are a number of possible models including the British Broadcasting Corporation, the Post Office, the University Grants Committee, the Manpower Services Commission.' But while many of the arguments in favour 'are attractive', the commission said, it was unpersuaded, offering a string of reasons against, including duplication of effort between the board and the department.[4]

Norman Fowler – who implemented the Griffiths report, the supervisory board and the management board – said in 2008 that 'by the end of my time [1987] I was basically in favour of a Health Service Commission, one that would have been one step away from the Department of Health. The Department had some extremely good advisers in it but the management knowledge, the direct experience of running and managing big organisations, was not actually a skill the department had. A health commission, with a separate board, separate chairman, separate chief executive, but with power, would have been the right way forward.

'I remember putting this once in conversation to Margaret Thatcher, and she thought about it and said "No, I don't think we can do that, they'll say we're just doing this as a prelude to privatising." And that, regrettably, is exactly what they would have said. I'm interested now to see that 10 or 15 years later [in 2008] it tends to be something that the Left of politics actually puts forward, as opposed to the Right.

'I hope it could successfully take some of the day-to-day politics and the day-to-day ministerial involvement out. It's certainly never going to be problem free because there are issues that come up which are obviously profoundly important, and there's no way round that. But if you ask me what is the best way of running an organisation as massive and complicated as the health service, I would not say that it was to have all the strands going back to the health department. It would be much better to have it run as you would run any other big organisation, but with that organisation being responsible to the minister.'[5]

Assorted Labour ministers, as we shall see in these interviews, also considered the idea. And it is one that, now that it is in existence, divides views among former health secretaries – but not on party lines.

It is just one of the issues we review as we explore their views around 'What is the role of the Secretary of State for Health?' and 'What should it be?'

Analysing the views of the former Secretaries of State for Health

What follows is an attempt to produce an analysis of the views, set out as edited transcripts in part 2 of this book, of the ten former health secretaries who so kindly agreed to be interviewed. It should be said that some were able to find more time for this than others, so the transcripts are not of equal length. Part 3 selects some key points on particular topics from across the interviews.

Although the broad framework of questions was the same – 'what is the role of the Secretary of State for Health? What should it be?' and so on – the conversations inevitably went off in many different directions with many different emphases. If time were no object, it would have been good to interview everyone again to put points each had raised to the others. Some of the views most often quoted in this section are from some of the more distant holders of the office. In part because it turns out that distance lends a greater perspective. And it should be stressed that what follows is one interpretation of their collective views. It would be possible to produce a very different one, drawing on the same interviews – which is one yet further encouragement to read them.

The transcripts contain the odd minor revelation. It is well known that Margaret Thatcher got cold feet in the summer of 1990 over the introduction in April 1991 of the purchaser/provider split, the so-called 'internal market' reform of the NHS. She had Ken Clarke and the department's senior executives in to Number 10 and was close to pulling them until Clarke made it clear that if she did so, he would resign.[3] What has not been known – or not known until Clarke's successor William Waldegrave recently published his memoir, *A Different Kind of Weather*[17] – is that when he took over five months before the reforms were to go live, she was prepared to ditch them again.

'She made it absolutely clear to me that if I wanted to cut the throat of all these reforms, that was fine as far as she was concerned,' Waldegrave says. Along with Duncan Nichol, the NHS chief executive, 'we persuaded her, and it was a matter of persuasion, that the thing made sense and it wasn't just Kenneth trying to cause trouble. But it was clear that she had no particular commitment to it at all.'

John Reid – the one health secretary since Ken Clarke we failed to engage with, so he is not represented here – famously went on to describe the Home Office as 'not fit for purpose' after he left health. Patricia Hewitt does not use that phrase. But she makes crystal clear her view that 'the leadership and capability within the department' was 'wholly inadequate' when she took over in 2005 – the unhappy period when the jobs of permanent secretary and chief executive of the NHS had been combined into one; when the NHS managed to achieve a significant overspend despite record levels of growth; and when a whole bunch of other things went wrong.

Indeed, the politicians' view that the department, or its management systems, was not always wholly up to the job is a recurring one. Clarke says that in the mid-1980s, and ahead of the Griffiths reforms 'there wasn't a management system worth the name'. Frank Dobson says of the late 1990s, 'it is not the fault of the top civil servants because they are displaying the characteristics that have been expected of them. But it tends to be staffed by people who produce a learned treatise on why the latest initiative has failed, rather than getting somebody who from the start makes sure it works' – though he very firmly excludes Alan Langlands, the NHS chief executive at the time, from that judgement. Hewitt's criticisms in the mid-2000s have already been referred to.

As the history above makes clear, the 'top of the office' arrangements in the department varied markedly over the years. But several health secretaries noted one unique feature of health – that, for many years, it had three permanent secretaries: the departmental permanent secretary, the chief medical officer and the NHS chief executive. In the days before an NHS chief executive it had two – a permanent secretary and a chief medical officer, who back then, was chief medical officer not just to the department but to the government as a whole.

That, of course, reflected the unique nature of the department's responsibilities. That it is clinicians – not just doctors but the whole range of clinicians – who deliver the

NHS on the ground, even if the influence of the medical profession collectively on health policy has declined over the years.

The status of these three permanent secretaries varied over time. Frank Dobson declares his surprise when he discovered that Ken Calman, the then chief medical officer, was not involved in policy discussions. He insisted he should be. Given the importance of clinicians in the NHS, Dobson says 'the idea that major issues are going to be discussed with the prime minister, and the chief medical officer isn't going to be there, seemed to me quite bizarre'. Alan Johnson, who aside from health was secretary of state for work and pensions, trade and industry, education and was home secretary to boot, says 'I have never known a department like it… so while the secretary of state was responsible, there was this triumvirate [at the top], well actually a quartet when you include me.' Only defence, with its armed forces chiefs of staff, who have an ultimate right to go direct to the prime minister, was reckoned in that way to be remotely comparable. Others noted how, by the 2000s, health was decidedly different to other departments, with most of the senior officials being NHS managers, rather than it being a classic Whitehall department.

Almost all the health secretaries had held ministerial jobs elsewhere. And despite health having the reputation of being the graveyard of political ambition, the vast majority had held other cabinet posts, often after, as well as before, being health secretary. Almost all said it was by far their most challenging job. The sense of stewardship. The sheer emotion that health generates. And the sense of accountability – and often for things they could not in reality be directly accountable for. All those contributed to the challenge, along with the permanent sense that a scandal or a crisis or just a huge public dispute could erupt at any moment. 'The toughest job I ever had,' says Clarke who, among other posts was chancellor, education and justice secretary, as well as being home secretary.

'Unbelievably demanding,' says Hewitt, who spoke of lying awake at 3am as she worried about the top of the office after Nigel Crisp's departure, a time when almost everyone who was senior was there in an acting capacity. The requirement to 'walk towards the guns' when things went wrong, as Virginia Bottomley puts it. 'You had to do the heavy lifting and walk towards the guns… [taking] responsibility for difficult news. I can't imagine how I survived at all!'

What is the role of the secretary of state?

At the most elementary level, all of the former health secretaries interviewed acknowledged the accountability they held for what is now a £100bn-a-year plus business. 'There is a custodian role to play, and an accountability to discharge,' as Alan Milburn puts it. Some put a heavier emphasis on the public health role, either from experience or desire. Andrew Lansley famously and ideally wanted to turn it into the department of public health, with the NHS being the responsibility only of a junior minister once he had set up his commissioning board – NHS England – as a separate statutory body with its annual rolling mandate. David Cameron, faced with one almighty row about Lansley's legislation and not wanting another, blocked that. Andy Burnham said that perhaps 'the primary duty' is to protect the public health, a view perhaps coloured by a pandemic of swine flu being declared by the World Health Organization three days into his tenure of the job.

But beyond that, there were many differences in emphasis. Some underlined the stewardship role. Others saw it as being the advocate for change. Clarke put this most clearly. 'The job is to lead change in response to changing demands and medical advances. To explain why you're making changes and try to get past the resistance you usually get from the staff, and certainly from the public – although I think people who work for the services have become less aggressively resistant to change.' Explaining that new requirements – the rise of the numbers of elderly with chronic conditions, for example – means changed services. 'You have to preside over change and explain it,' he says.

But Waldegrave shrewdly observed that the job also 'depends on whether you think the system, at any given time, is in need of policy reform. I came to think it did.' As, clearly, did Clarke, Milburn and Lansley, while others – Bottomley, Dorrell, Hewitt, Johnson – were, broadly speaking, there to implement, or to enhance, or to adapt a broad thrust of policy that had already been agreed.

Dobson said the job was to implement any manifesto promises because the failure to do that 'is the most damaging part of politics'. But it was then to 'try to help all the people involved do their jobs as well as they would like to do them, by removing obstructions and lunacies out of their way and really trying to make the system work, rather than constantly tinkering and pissing around with it.' Though he observes that was 'an alien concept as far as the Blairite Downing Street was concerned, who wanted an initiative every 20 minutes'.

Which brings up a subject rarely discussed – the relationship between the health secretary and the prime minister. Clarke's relationship with Thatcher was famously rumbustious – but, as he has said elsewhere, both liked to make their minds up by furious argument. Stephen Dorrell said the role of the health secretary is determined to some extent by the views of the voters, those of the incumbent, and those of the prime minister. The views of the incumbent will vary – 'I have a very strong view about what the role ought to be… which is that you're not responsible for making all the decisions'. The voters matter because they expect the secretary of state to be accountable. And the prime minister, 'because for the prime minister, the health secretary is a kind of risk manager. They only have one objective for a health secretary, which is to keep the NHS out of the newspapers… That's what leads health secretaries into what I think is a blind alley, which is believing that risk management is best delivered by more control.'

Alan Johnson was also among those who felt that part of the job was to manage the prime minister and try to keep him or her out of it. 'There were things I didn't want to do that Gordon [Brown] insisted we did like free prescriptions for patients with cancer.' Not, he felt, a good use of the money when the vast bulk of prescriptions are dispensed free and there is an annual cap available, currently £104, on how much any individual pays. There was – is – often a search for some eye-catching announcement, driven from Number 10. And that has happened under government of all colours. 'They want to say something on health – so what can you fish up?' as Johnson puts it.

Patricia Hewitt says: 'It would help if you had prime ministers who had thought more about health policy and the NHS, and how the two were best approached, before they became prime minister. And that then informed their choice of health secretary. The chance of that would be a fine thing! Not very likely to happen.'

Clarke is most blunt about it. 'When a prime minister gets panicked and starts intervening, I think it is the duty of the secretary of state to get him or her out of the way. Most of them don't have the time to know anything about how the health service is run.' If the health secretary ducks when a crisis occurs, 'then suddenly the prime minister will just insist on going to Rotherham to start making pronouncements on what they're doing or something, and you can't have that. They start stamping their little foot and going for photo opportunities, and trying to get command and control – which they can't.' Dobson too sought to resist 'an initiative every 20 minutes' even though his period is seen by many as one of the heights of an attempt to run the NHS by command and control.

What should the role be?
There was complete unanimity that ministers should not be involved in the day-to-day nitty-gritty management of the NHS. As Alan Johnson put it – pretty much on behalf of all

of them – 'I don't think when a bed pan falls on the floor in Tredegar it should echo around Whitehall any more.' But after that, there was a wide range of views.

First over how that might be achieved. And second over how far ministers should be and in practice can be distanced from broader operational matters – in other words, over how far it is possible, in the real world, to separate policy from implementation, and thus policy from operations and management.

Frank Dobson was the one who declared that – up to a point – 'I have no problem with command and control. It is part of the secretary of state's job.' He cites a range of examples, including his own interventions to get the meningitis C vaccine sorted, to get digital hearing aids introduced and to provide more modern prostheses. He also describes deciding how NHS Direct would be trialled, and then insisting that the civil servant who had got it up and running, but who had been promoted and moved elsewhere, should be brought back.

'It may have helped that before I was an MP I worked for the Central Electricity Generating Board and I had to organise things and get them done. I worked at making things work before I was an MP. So that may have coloured my view.

'So my attitude to policy was, "Okay, right that's the policy, well how do we implement it? Because there isn't a Rolls Royce machine that is going to implement it".

In Dobson's view, the split of NHS England into a statutorily independent commissioning board is, quite simply, 'bollocks… the idea that the NHS is going to be this independent organisation, without political interference, and this, that and the other, is just rubbish and it has proved to be just rubbish.

'Every time anything crops up the [current] secretary of state intervenes and blames somebody else. Because this distancing has meant that he can blame somebody else but not accept any blame himself. Which I think was probably the object of the exercise. But it doesn't mean that there isn't political interference... he clearly is interfering all the time.

'I think the person who takes the decisions should carry the can and the person who carries the can should take the decisions. There isn't any way in the end... that people will not expect the health secretary to be responsible, and take the blame when things go wrong.'

Stephen Dorrell is no more in favour of a statutorily independent board, although in less colourful language. 'When people said to me what did I think about the coalition setting up an independent board, I used to say, "Well, I am the person who abolished the last one!"'.

The NHS Policy Board (see above) was created by Ken Clarke, although interestingly its role does not feature highly in his memory. It sat above what was then the NHS Management Executive, partly to provide some strategic oversight over the 1991 reforms as they came in, and partly to provide some distance. It was, notably, not independent of ministers, and not statutory – any more than was the management executive, a key part of whose function in the eyes of Duncan Nichol, the then chief executive, was 'separating the role of managers from ministers'.

Waldegrave revamped the policy board. But he faced what he says is the 'inherent difficulty of trying to separate the management from policy... I didn't want anybody else, perhaps wrongly, to be chairman of the policy board. So I made myself the chairman. It was implicitly saying that the secretary of state should not just be policy, but should also be an executive. Perhaps I shouldn't have chaired it. But then this is the inherent difficulty of the whole thing – is it possible, in any business or in any organisation, truly to separate policy from execution? I certainly thought then that to see the policy through, I had to retain the strategic control of what was happening...'

Virginia Bottomley saw the policy board as being 'outside advisers'. It met in series with the bi-monthly meetings of the then very powerful regional chairs. It might, she says, 'have been very useful when the NHS reforms were being set up. But creating agendas for both became ridiculous. You tell me Stephen abolished it. Well, he was completely right.'

Dorrell says he attended the board when he was a junior health minister and Clarke was health secretary, while personally 'not really getting it' – what it was for. 'I think I cancelled two, or maybe even three meetings, of this assembly at short notice, thinking I had better ways of spending my time. And it became an embarrassment. It had got to point where it either had to meet or I had to abolish it. So I abolished it.'

As already noted, Dorrell's view is that the health secretary should not be responsible for every decision. 'What you are responsible for is outcomes and structures and incentives. You are responsible for the effect of the decisions, but you're not responsible for the decisions themselves.' He agreed that he sought to behave more like the chair of the board of a company than the chief executive – and, in not only this author's judgement, but in the eyes of others, he is the health secretary who came closest to that. Alan Langlands, who was chief executive at the time, met him, outside crises, once a week – to compare notes and get a lead where he needed it, or when Dorrell wanted to give him one. He was a 'non-interventionist chairman,' Langlands has recorded. 'A big-picture chairman. He was interested in ideas and did not want to get bogged down in detail.'[9] This does not mean that Dorrell did not introduce change. A significant and modernising revamp of the GP contract, for example, happened on his watch.

But, Dorrell says, 'all this stuff about creating independent decision making and getting the health service out of politics blah, blah, blah… Well, that's exactly the same speech that we used to make in favour of the health authorities that were statutorily independent. They existed in statute. They had responsibilities defined in statute. So what's changed?

'I've never quite believed these parallels with the BBC or the Bank of England's independence. The BBC is completely different. Voters don't need to be persuaded that journalism should be independent of politics. They don't want politicians interfering, so that one's easy to explain. The Bank of England is trickier. But essentially it only has one target, which is much easier than the NHS which is full of competing desirable outcomes. I was an advocate of an independent Bank. But we don't yet know, in truth, how the voters will react if inflation gets out of control because the Bank has got its interest rate policy seriously wrong. When we get to that, then we'll know how well the voters take to the principle of an independent Bank of England. Will they really accept that Mark Carney has an existence in their lives independent of George Osborne when Mark Carney or his successor bogs up and George says it's nothing to do with him? That will be the test.'

The Independent Reconfiguration Panel has helped, he says. But in practice 'it has reflected the will of ministers at the time – to allow a process to take place and to give themselves excuses. As far as voters are concerned, the ministers were responsible for the reconfiguration that they'd allowed to happen. You can't legislate away responsibility.'

That point seems irrefutable in a tax-funded system. When Mid-Staffordshire first broke, Alan Johnson had the entire top team in his room and turned to David Nicholson as the NHS chief executive. The two agreed that there was no alternative but to get rid of the chair and the chief executive. But Mid-Staffordshire, famously, had just become a foundation trust, and Bill Moyes, Monitor's chief executive and chair, piped up and asked, in one sense entirely correctly, 'under what legal authority, secretary of state, are you going to do that?' – given that under Labour's legislation it was Monitor who approved foundation trust status and had the power to replace boards and chief executives. Johnson replied: 'Look, this is what we are going to do. I've spoken to the prime minister about it. I'm up in the House tomorrow answering questions about it. I am the Secretary of State for Health. And I'm responsible. And that's what we are going to do. I don't give a damn what the legislation says.'

In his interview, Johnson confirms that story. 'Now, politically, it would be very nice if you could get away with it and say, "That's yours. That's your can of worms." Moyes was probably right that the legislation said he was responsible, Johnson says. 'But I told him, you know, "Piss off. I'm dealing with this."… You are the secretary of state. There is public money going in there. You are responsible.'

Personally, he says, 'there was absolutely no way that I would have set up this huge quango, NHS England, to protect ministers from that. There was no way I would have pursued that because it was never going to work. Parliamentarians aren't going to put up with being told, "Nothing to do with us. Write to NHS England".'

The lesson that has to be drawn from this is that behaviour trumps legislation. And arguably that can be seen in the time of Jeremy Hunt, the first health secretary actually to operate with Lansley's statutorily independent board in place. For example, it was Hunt in 2013 and 2014 who decided to inject extra cash for winter pressures; who issued guidance on hospital car parking charges and hospital food; and who personally called hospital chief executives whose A&E performance was slipping – though Hunt says this was in order to understand what was causing that, not to berate them.* By early 2015 Oliver Letwin and Eric Pickles were members of a cabinet committee fretting over the NHS's day-to-day performance in the run-up to the general election.

A tortured debate could be held over whether the first three of these examples are matters of policy or of implementation – an issue to which we will return.

---

* Speaking at the Nuffield Trust Summit in 2015 he said: 'If you speak to any of the chief executives I have spoken to about discussions about A&E they would say, I hope, that it is not a call from the boss holding them to account, it is a call from the health secretary to try to understand what the pressures are and how we can help more than we are currently doing.'

But even Andrew Lansley – the high priest of the 'depoliticisation of the NHS' and who enters a fierce defence of his reforms in his interview – concedes that ministers are still intervening on operational issues, whatever the legislation says. 'I [do] think they're still intervening – of course they are – but it will get harder and harder over time.' Of Hunt's actions, he says 'he knows he shouldn't'. But Lansley argues that some of these apparent interventions are 'stuff which NHS England has in practice decided and ministers are badging for political reasons'. Which, in itself, begs the question of where the divide lies.

Jeremy Hunt was not interviewed for this piece. But elsewhere, when challenged that he has been highly interventionist, he said: 'any health secretary of any government, with a democratic mandate, has the right to decide on a few priorities. The areas that they think most need change. So I have picked on the areas that I want to focus on. Improving compassionate care – the Francis agenda. Transforming the way we deal with dementia. The technology revolution, and out-of-hospital care. These are areas that I am particularly focusing on. And I think any secretary of state would have those priorities.

'And I do not think you could do a job like mine without deciding on a few priorities and focusing on how to change those. But I think the day-to-day micro-management is something that happens less. And I think we have a system that is evolving – it is new. And a system with a mandate where a vast majority of NHS delivery is left to NHS England to deliver as it sees fit and in accordance with what is in the mandate. And it will evolve.'

But 'I do not think it was ever going to be the case that the secretary of state could step right back.' Asked if that meant that the absolutely pure model of depoliticisation outlined in Lansley's white paper will never be achieved, he said: 'I think we are evolving in that way. But we also have to recognise that we are a democracy. And people want to hold people like me, rightly, accountable for over £100bn of public money, and so there are always going to be times when the health secretary has to involve themselves in operational issues.'*

Johnson's view that ministers are responsible does not mean that he believes there are not ways in which some of the politics can be taken out of the NHS, or at least diluted – and that there are ways that some management decisions can indeed be distanced from ministers. All ministers quoted NICE. Johnson used the Independent Reconfiguration Panel that Reid had set up. While, like a wise, politician, he 'never said never', he did say: 'I can foresee no circumstances in which I would intervene' against its recommendations. And he stuck to that. He also set up the Cooperation and Competition Panel. Its non-statutory task was, in Labour's new world of choice and competition, to advise on competition issues when they arose in the NHS. Johnson admits that choice and competition 'never really got my juices flowing' as the key driver for change. But he says of the panel, 'I can't remember much about it. It did its stuff and I don't remember it ever causing us any problems, which is a measure of its success. And now Andrew Lansley has turned it into this monster through legislation, so now we have competition lawyers sitting in the corner every time two hospitals talk to each other.'

Ken Clarke may have set up both a supervisory and a policy board, and indeed had packed the NHS Management Executive off to Leeds in an attempt to separate the management out more from the politicians. But he is deeply unconvinced that a statutory board will seriously depoliticise the NHS. 'I did used to tell Andrew that his belief that you could depoliticise the whole thing by having this statutory separation for NHS England was highly desirable but very naïve. I said, "You will still find you're in

* Speaking at the Nuffield Trust Summit, February 2014.

the middle of rows about bedpans dropped in wards". He did try to go to huge lengths to detach himself totally from a lot of decision making.

'Every secretary of state has been trying to depoliticise the daily management of the system, detach themselves from it, because the political arguments are ludicrously unhelpful.

'But faced with huge petitions and MPs lobbying you in the House of Commons you will never entirely get away with saying "This is nothing to do with me. I have no powers over this." I think we're a long way from ever achieving that. But we'll see how it goes.'

If Johnson's view is that he would never have set up an independent NHS England, Labour ministers in fact looked at the idea of at least some sort of independent board several times. Gordon Brown trailed the idea in public, ahead of taking over from Tony Blair. Andy Burnham, Johnson's successor, examined it. 'The board was discussed at the point of transition [between Tony Blair and Gordon Brown] and Gordon's team got interested in it. But when we thought about it, it quickly dropped away when you thought about the implications. So we backed off. You simply cannot have £100bn-worth of public money without democratic accountability. I remember people saying, "You couldn't have MPs writing and the secretary of state saying 'Oh, don't ask me'", which is kind of what happens now.

'If politics has a respectable role, it's obviously in providing accountability for taxation. And if that doesn't apply in respect of the NHS, then what does it apply to?'

Furthermore, Burnham says, he had a similar clash with Monitor to Johnson's when he discovered that the chief executive and chair at Mid Staffordshire were still interim appointments. 'I asked "Why haven't we got the best in the NHS in there now?" and was told, "Oh well, [it is] Monitor – they don't want to put anybody in. And you set up Monitor and it's your foundation trust reform." I basically at that point realised that it just doesn't work in that scenario. You have to be able to override systems, and the requirements for public safety and good governance means that politicians will occasionally have to step in.'

He adds however that 'I do think it's good if secretaries of state don't get too involved' while adding that it is 'a very hard balance.' He would not, he says, get rid of NHS England, though he would probably 'pull it back in some way'. That 'doesn't mean that you then pull everything back in. The chief executive, who was based in the department, probably could sit outside of the department and that is a healthy thing – that arm's-length arrangement. It's not about saying we just get rid of NHS England. There is a respectable case to be made for running the NHS separate from the government structure, outside the department.' But 'there is a debate to be had about statutory independence.'

In Milburn's time, an independent board was not on the agenda: there was far too much to do in getting the NHS Plan up and running. But he favours in theory the distinction between strategy (something for ministers) and operations (something for clinicians and managers). 'You separate yourself from the operations, and deal with the strategic. That is the theory. The only thing that buggers it is the practice!' he says.

The whole thrust of his reforms – giving hospitals a greater statutory underpinning of independence through foundation trust status than NHS trusts had enjoyed, creating the first version of Monitor, introducing a tariff, and the independent sector treatment centres, along with the policies of choice and competition – was about that, he argues. 'Setting overall objectives, aligning resources behind objectives, sticking to strategy, and keeping out of operations, broadly.'

Organisationally and architecturally, he says, the NHS is a very different model to 1948 and the years of the 1970s. 'But culturally and politically, it isn't. We changed some architecture but we haven't changed culture and we haven't changed politics. That's why it's really hard. Because every time there's a problem – guess what? Some poor bugger – whether it's me or Ken Clarke or Jeremy Hunt – will get dragged to the despatch box and have to answer for themselves.

'In the end, the only thing that can break that is politics. Politics is the trap. And the only thing that can break it is politics. I'm afraid there is not a surfeit of politicians who think that their historical purpose, having got power, is somehow to give it away. That's what you've got to do. That's what, in a sense, Ken was trying to do. That, in the end, with foundation trusts and markets and all that stuff, is what I was trying to do. That's an uncompleted journey…

'So you ask does that mean that I think the idea of NHS England as a statutorily independent body is something that I broadly approve? Well, I think it is a stepping stone. I mean it's a monstrous bureaucracy. But it is definitely part of that.'

Patricia Hewitt too looked seriously at some sort of independent board. 'Although the Lansley reforms have created the most appalling mess,' she says, 'and a lot of good people and capability have been weakened or destroyed in the process, there is also, I think, a very strong team in Simon Stevens [Chief Executive of NHS England] and those around him. The independence, or greater degree of independence, of NHS England, and the very clear responsibility that they have got for the NHS is, I think, helpful.

'I was actually quite attracted by the idea of an NHS commissioning role. I had very interesting discussions, both with my special advisers and with officials about it. And they just said, "It's impossible. You cannot give away responsibility for £100bn. The secretary of state has to be responsible to parliament for that." Now, actually the secretary of state remains accountable to parliament for it, even under the 2012 Act. But I felt very strongly that there were far too many issues, including clinical issues, coming onto my desk, in a very Nye

Bevan way, really. The bedpan dropping in Tredegar. It was quite ludicrous. And you needed an NHS leadership.

'But the creation of the commissioning board – which in a sense was a logical next step from recreating the split between the permanent secretary and the NHS chief executive – I think that does have some merit.

'The distinction between policy and implementation is never as clear as people sometimes pretend. If you make policy without understanding both the constraint of implementation and the possibilities of implementation… then you will get policy wrong. Therefore there is absolutely a risk, if you split it in the way that the commissioning board does, then you weaken the input of implementation into policy. You have to guard against that.'

But, she says, 'The Five Year Forward View is essentially a letter which says that "with incredible effort on efficiency, and productivity gains, and some big changes in terms of behaviour, and prevention, etc. we can close a large part of [the financial gap]. But we cannot close it all".

'I think that's really powerful. And it would be quite hard to do that with the chief executive within the department. Probably impossible. They could do it privately, to the health secretary. But that's a very different matter from doing it publicly with the authority of the board behind you. Of course there are disadvantages. But that strikes me as quite a big advantage, particularly in the highly uncertain political environment that the UK finds itself in.'

Conclusions

So what emerges from this? Well, everyone save the man himself was withering about Andrew Lansley's 2012 Act. 'That enormous Act was just hubris' Ken Clarke says, even as he adds that 'I'm the only politician in the House of Commons who says that Andrew Lansley's reforms, on the whole, seem to be quite beneficial, and once they settle down they'll have a good effect.' Lansley, almost needless to say, is deeply sanguine about it all. Despite the language in his white paper, it wasn't, he says, about 'removing politicians'. It was about 'at least restricting them. Trying to hamstring the politicians a bit. Of course, we will only know in 10 years' time if it's worked.'

But what also emerges is that there is in fact both cross-party agreement, and cross-party disagreement, about the merits of a statutorily independent board. On both the Labour and Conservative side, some see advantages in it, some not. Clarke says: 'The reason I think it is working so far is that the board [NHS England] is not actually asserting itself as a rival centre of power. It is actually giving a clinician-led – apparently clinician-led – lead to policy making.'

It will work, he says, so long as there is a very close working relationship between the chief executive and the minister – something that he argues applies equally to the independence of the Bank of England. As Clarke quintessentially puts it, so long as there is a genuinely close working relationship 'then he [the governor or the Chief Executive of NHS England] can be as independent as he likes, so long as he is not doing anything that the secretary of state is getting too upset about!'

Almost all the health secretaries were clear that the distinctions between strategy and operations, between policy and implementation, and between strategy, policy and management are, quite simply, not as clear as the policy wonks like to make them in their beautiful organograms of how the NHS is meant to function at any given time. It's a muddled world. There is 'the inherent difficulty', as Waldegrave puts it, of whether it is possible 'in any business or in any organisation, truly to separate policy from execution?'

All the health secretaries agreed that the personality of the incumbent, and the way they choose to operate, or the way they instinctively operate, matters – whatever the legislation says. From Virginia Bottomley (though she was far from the only one) being obsessed about the media coverage – in her case because she cared about its impact on the staff and patients; to Stephen Dorrell's more chair of the board-like behaviour; to Frank Dobson 'wandering up and down the ministerial corridor in my stockinged feet, like the non-executive chairman'; to the mighty reforming drive of Clarke and Milburn (whatever your views on the merit of those changes); to the gentle, humour-laced, reassurance that Alan Johnson brought to the job, along with a hint of steel. In each case, behaviour matters. It trumps legislation.

And, for all the fact that most of the changes that directly affect patients in the NHS are clinically driven – by medical advance or by evidence that shows there is a better way of organising services, or by patients' views of the service, or by changing clinical needs – the main policy changes to the infrastructure and the incentives in the NHS come from politicians. The guardians of the taxpayer's pound. Or at least they do in the politicians' eyes.

Milburn says: 'Now I might have been either a terrible secretary of state, or I might have been just an aberration, but reform didn't come from the system.

'Why do people, whether it's right or wrong, why do they now rather, through rose tinted glasses, look back fondly on my time? Why? Because they feel that there was clarity. There was energy. There was determination. And there was shared mission because actually we were smart enough, I hope, to construct a shared view of what we wanted to do. It was because politics was driving it. So I think you've just got to be a bit careful with this debate because it can very easily turn into – "if only the politicians got out of this, everything would be wonderful".

'If they do, fuck all would happen because what do systems do? What do bureaucracies do? They don't change. By definition they don't change so you've got to have a shock. Politics should be able to provide shock.' Clarke certainly provided one. So did Lansley, though as the other health secretaries make clear, that was another matter.

Dorrell says: 'You've heard me say it, times without number, that actually health policy hasn't changed. Frank Dobson would like to have changed it and wasn't able to. But apart from him, no health secretary has wanted to change policy since 1991, which is the day when it really did change. We used to have a provider-led system; we now have a commissioner-led system. That is different. But it's the last time anybody fundamentally changed health policy. The question lies between the concept and the execution. That's where the story is – and the disability, the powerlessness of commissioners, is the result of consistent execution failure. But that's hardly surprising when successive governments have reorganised the commissioner side every five years. Well, of course it doesn't work if you change it every five years.'

There is a lot of truth in that. But as already noted, Waldegrave's first observation was that 'the job of the Secretary of State for Health depends on whether you think the system, at any given time, is in need of policy reform'.

Andy Burnham says: 'It all depends on the context, it really does. I would encourage you to think about this, because every secretary of state operates in a different context. I'll give you two things I know very, very well. Number one was a financial meltdown, which you remember well. It was one of those things where the system almost collectively loses its way. It does need to be, one by one, brought back into a proper financial position. I saw Patricia do that, and it was successful.

'The second example from my time was swine flu… people think about Mid Staffs. But the thing that was most immediate for me was swine flu. I remember being in the secretary of state's office, asking, "What does it mean?". They explained the arrangements that were going to kick in – 'Gold Command' and all this kind of thing. I remember David Nick [Nicholson] winking at me saying, "We're in command and control mode now." It was a self-reflective, self-deprecating joke. But it was important. We did have to go into that mode… and people wanted us to. Very clear advice, instructions to PCTs, instructions through NHS Direct. We did have to have some negotiations with the GPs. But once that had been done, it had to be implemented in full. In those early days when the pandemic had been declared, it was pretty serious. Although it turned out not be as bad as people feared, it was pretty frightening for a while.

'When the Lansley reforms came along, we said, "what are you going to do in a similar situation?" The beauty of the secretary of state's power is that it is there. Yes, in ordinary times you would expect an individual to use it with a very light touch and permissive feel. That would be the ideal. But there will be moments where, because it's there, you can use it to its full benefit to protect the public.'

Or to put it another way, in Virginia Bottomley's words, there is an irregular cycle to these things – how far management responsibility can be devolved when policy is changing. She came, she says, 'to like the idea of an independent board… some distance from ministers for the NHS'. And some distance, in one form or another, was something that all those interviewed favoured.

'But there are different times in politics' she says, 'and it does go in cycles'. There is a truth in that which she did not mention but which can, for example, be traced back to Enoch Powell's hospital plan and his 'water towers' speech, or to Barbara Castle's promotion of the need to do something about the 'Cinderella services'.

'Sometimes,' Bottomley says, 'you want a window breaker and sometimes you want a glazier. Ken was a window breaker and he was brilliant. But after that you get William Waldegrave who was a glazier. And my job, after the election [in 1992] was that we'd got some trusts and fundholders up and running and my task was to get all of that beyond a tipping point. Quieten it all down. Show them you care. And then a new set of problems will arrive and you need a Ken to break the windows again.' Just as Milburn did.

For all that, however, there is a long-run journey here that can be seen to be playing out. The service moved from being an essentially *administered* one in the 1950s and 1960s to a *managed* one in the 1980s as ministers searched for levers that they could pull so that democratically elected politicians could be more confident that nationally expressed policy was implemented on the ground. In the 1990s, more *market-like mechanisms* (though nothing like a proper market) were instituted in an attempt to move away from that directly managed service to what Labour later called a more 'self-improving' one.

Put another way, the long-run story is that as the NHS moved through these three stages ministers first sought more control over the management of the service then tried, far from always successfully, to give it away.

That long-run period did indeed involve genuine attempts by ministers to distance themselves from the management of the service – even as, paradoxically, those very changes not only made command and control more possible, it also sometimes required it. The laying down of market rules, for example, or the introduction of independent sector treatment centres as an attempt to boost competition.

It is also impossible to ignore secular trends here. For example, the arrival of information technology – essentially computing and email. First computing made it possible to collect more data to analyse and understand and use to influence performance. And then email provided a speed of communication up and down the NHS that was unthinkable at any time until the late 1990s. Both proved powerful centripetal forces.

But, as Dorrell says, 'it's all about pushing it down. If you don't do that, you have a bunch of disempowered managers.'

Or, as Clarke puts it, 'every secretary of state has been trying to depoliticise the daily management of the system, detach themselves from it, because the political arguments are ludicrously unhelpful,' even if, as Hunt observes, 'people want to hold people like me, rightly, accountable, for over £100bn of public money, and so there are always going to be times when the health secretary has to involve themselves in operational issues'.* So the question remains. Where does the balance lie? And is it in the right place right now?

But that's my interpretation of what the health secretaries said. Read the interviews, and form your own view.

Nicholas Timmins

---

* Speaking at the Nuffield Trust Summit, February 2014.

References

1. *Nursing Times* 12 June 1948; cited in Webster C. *Bevan on the NHS*. Wellcome Unit for the History of Medicine, 1991.

2. Klein R. *The new politics of the NHS*. Fifth Edition. Oxford: Radcliffe Publishing, 2006.

3. Timmins N. *The five giants: A biography of the Welfare State*. HarperCollins, 2001.

4. Royal Commission on the National Health Service. Cmnd 7615. HMSO, 1979.

5. Nuffield Trust. *Rejuvenate or retire? Views of the NHS at 60*. Nuffield Trust, 2008.

6. Report of the committee of enquiry into the cost of the national health service. (Chairman: CW Guillebaud.) Cmd 9663. London: HMSO, 1956.

7. Department of Health. *Working for Patients*, Cm 555, January 1989.

8. Griffiths R. *Report of the NHS Management Inquiry*. February 1983.

9. Edwards B, Fall M. *The executive years of the NHS*. Nuffield Trust. Radcliffe Publishing, 2005.

10. *The Independent* 25 January 1994.

11. Hansard. *HC Deb 21 October 1993 vol 230 cc398-412.*

12. Banks T. *Review of the wider Department of Health*. Department of Health, 1994.

13. Greer S, Jarman H. *The Department of Health and the Civil Service: From Whitehall to Department of Delivery to Where?* Nuffield Trust, 2006.

14. Department of Health. *Equity and Excellence: Liberating the NHS* Cm 7881 July 2010.

15. Healthcare on the Brink of a Cultural Revolution. *Financial Times*, 16 January 2011.

16. Timmins N. *Never again: The story of the Health and Social Care Act 2012*. Institute for Government and the King's Fund, 2012.

17. Waldegrave W. *A different kind of weather*. Constable, 2015.

Part 2:

*In their own words:
interviews with former
Secretaries of State for Health*

'I closed more hospitals than most people had hot dinners.'

Kenneth Clarke
July 1988 – November 1990

Rt Hon Kenneth Clarke QC was Minister of Health from 1982 to 1985 and Secretary of State for Health from July 1988 to November 1990. His other posts include Chancellor of the Exchequer, Home Secretary and Education Secretary.

The job is to lead change in response to changing demands and medical advances. To explain why you're making the changes and try to get past the resistance you usually get from the staff, and certainly from the public. I think actually people who work for the service have become less aggressively resistant to change. Their trade unions haven't. But the people in the service have become less aggressively resistant to the fact that the patient, and the care that is provided, move on all the time.

I always joke with Jeremy [Hunt] that being minister of health is a political deathbed in most western democracies. In every western democracy, health is the most controversial subject that politicians encounter, because it's so emotional and there are such tensions and competing interests. It's also one of the most important. I must say that he seems to be surviving quite well.

When I was first there, I learned about the health service when I was minister of state, when it was run in a comically bad fashion. The problem is that there wasn't a management system worth the name. There was next to no management information of any kind, no one knew what the devil we were spending the money on, and the whole thing was dominated by political campaigning.

You tend to forget what the atmosphere was like in the 1980s, when the politics of every large organisation, not just the health service, was dominated by industrial relations. It was probably true of half the big businesses in the country that two-thirds of the time of the chief executive was spent on industrial relations.

It wasn't command and control, although there was this mad illusion that I was supposed to command and control it.

It wasn't command and control, although there was this mad illusion that I was supposed to command and control it.

That I was sitting there in the middle with all these thousands of staff. I think I was the first to point out that it was the largest employer in Europe apart from the Red Army.

You were of course held responsible every time anybody dropped a bedpan, and somehow you had a huge administrative structure, which ensured that you controlled all this. It was hopeless. It was a gruesome, self-perpetuating bureaucracy, riddled with vested interests. It was collapsing.

One of my first introductions to the service was that I had to go to close a maternity hospital in Clement Freud's constituency [the Isle of Ely]… A great demonstration took place, and they were moving the babies inside to try to give me the impression there were more than there were. I met the local grand consultants, the obstetricians, who told me ferociously – addressing a minister of state in an absolutely James Robertson Justice way – that I had got to close this place. And they had all agreed that they were not going to accept any more referrals to it. 'It was dangerous!' – and they had a better facility in some local East Anglian town.

So I said: 'Come out with me and say that to all these women and these television cameras outside who are waving babies at me.' And they refused. Absolutely refused. And it turned out they had not shared this opinion with anybody but me and the doctors from whom they were refusing to accept referrals. One of them said, 'That is your job, we are not prepared to do that.' That is a silly story, but it is a true story. It was my first introduction to the fact that some of the medical profession had no time at all for those who did manage the service, but were not prepared to accept the slightest responsibility for managing any change.

In fact I closed more hospitals than most people had hot dinners – old Victorian workhouses which were called 'geriatric hospitals' but which suddenly became centres of clinical excellence when their closure was proposed.

When I was minister of health I did do some command and control. Trying to get some control over the manpower and get some efficiency into the system. We did have the regional chairmen, and the chairs of the district health authorities. Refusing to reappoint them was the only lever I had, and the one I continued to pull all the time. I gradually got rid of the ones [the chairs] who used to go on strike with the staff and stand on the picket lines, and got in people who were good, local businessmen – not very political, most of them. That was regarded as a real novelty. I used to describe them as my 'health cabinet'.

And then Margaret [Thatcher] brought in Roy Griffiths. I resented him being there at first. There I was clattering about, contracting out this and manpowering that in an attempt to get some management into the service, and here's this bloke they want to bring in to spend 12 months doing a study. Some businessman from a food store who is in some vague way going to work alongside me. In fact, Roy produced a very good report. My reluctance about it turned out to be a terrible mistake. Roy knew 10 times more about management than I did, and he was right. He came to broadly the same conclusions I had come to.

The service didn't have any managers. There was great resistance to having managers. And there are still all these silly clichéd populist comments that always get wheeled out before elections about getting rid of managers – as if this giant organisation doesn't need any management!

When I came back as Secretary of State for Health in 1988 we introduced the purchaser/provider split – and, of course, there were flaming rows and battles about that. What we were trying to do was introduce a system that was much more responsive to demand at the local level, that was led by patient demands, and where the people providing the service could respond to them in the best way within the finite resources that were going to be available to them.

Every secretary of state insists they made the most significant change, but I, like all the others, arrogantly believe that the purchaser/provider split was the most significant change after 1948. I always knew it would be imperfect when we introduced it and it would need to be refined and changed as it went along. But it has lasted and been continued apart from a slight pause under Frank Dobson who made the terrible mistake of abolishing GP fundholding, which GPs, at least in my patch, still tell me they bitterly regret. But after 18 months Tony Blair decided that appointing Frank was a mistake and the reforms resumed under Alan Milburn who went a lot further than I would ever have got away with, or dared. I was a great fan of Alan Milburn when he was health secretary. So purchaser/provider has survived, but in a much more sophisticated way. And actually Andrew Lansley has

I believe the purchaser/ provider split was the most significant change after 1948.

succeeded in localising it yet further. Clinicians do own it now. There is less resistance to change.

NHS England has produced a plan, admittedly only sketching an outline, of how to tackle the changes that come with an ageing population and both political parties have signed up to it. Simon Stevens advocates local variation and you are beginning to get the change coming from the bottom up. It's early days and it needs to develop, but I think it is working quite well now, after everybody disowned it. I'm the only politician in the House of Commons who says that Andrew Lansley's reforms, on the whole, seem to be quite beneficial, and once they settle down they'll have a good effect.

The scale of disruption in introducing them was ridiculous. That enormous bill [the Health and Social Care Bill] was just hubris. I argued to him that he didn't need a bill. That all of it, certainly almost all of it, could have been done within his existing powers. But he built it up into this monumental refounding of the NHS. The reason Andrew failed was because he couldn't explain it. He got immersed in all the technicalities and even I couldn't follow what he was going on about. He needed some broad-brush stuff, instead of which he immersed himself in the detail so that nobody understood it, and everybody got fearful that some dreadful change was being made. It was over-elaborated. But the underlying point was okay.

So I supported Andrew Lansley's reforms. But I did used to tell Andrew that his belief that you could depoliticise the whole thing by having this statutory separation for NHS England was highly desirable but very naïve. I said, 'You will still find you're in the middle of rows about bedpans dropped in wards.' He did try to go to huge lengths to detach himself totally from a lot of decision making.

Every secretary of state has been trying to depoliticise the daily management of the system, detach themselves from it, because the political arguments are ludicrously unhelpful.

But faced with huge petitions and MPs lobbying you in the

House of Commons you will never entirely get away with saying, 'This is nothing to do with me. I have no powers over this.' I think we're a long way from ever achieving that. But we'll see how it goes.

The reason I think it is working so far is that the board [NHS England] is not actually asserting itself as a rival centre of power. It is actually giving a clinician-led – apparently clinician-led – lead to policy making. Going back to my maternity hospital story, this time the service appears, to the general public and to the politicians, to be identifying a priority and offering to deliver it.

I very much trust that Jeremy [Hunt] and Simon Stevens have a very close working relationship. I'm a great believer in an independent Bank of England, but one thing an independent Bank of England requires is a very close relationship with the chancellor. The chancellor and the governor of the Bank of England have got to sit down, once a week, over a lunch, with perhaps the odd private secretary, and nobody else there. I didn't have an independent Bank of England, unfortunately, because John [Major] wouldn't let me. But I did run this arrangement with Eddie George [the governor of the day]. The chancellor has sometimes got to bang on about the political realities of what you can and cannot do, and the governor of the Bank has got to bang on about what he thinks the consequences will and will not be. The two of you have got to have an extremely good working relationship. Then he can be as independent as he likes, so long as he is not doing anything that the secretary of state is getting too upset about! I'm sure George Osborne and Mark Carney are in and out of each other's offices all the time, not least because the other can screw up what you want to do. And NHS England will fail if they have a secretary of state who's impotent but furious, and not able to defend it.

Jeremy has got involved in some operational detail because he didn't have Andrew's belief that he could avoid it, and he's right. People will regard you as a complete idiot if you don't, and then suddenly the prime minister will just insist on going to Rotherham to start making pronouncements on what they're doing or something, and you can't have that. They start stamping their little foot and going for photo opportunities, and trying to get command and control, which they can't.

When a prime minister gets panicked and starts intervening, I think it is the duty of the secretary of state to get him or her out of the way. Most of them don't have the time to know anything about how the health service is run. It goes back to what I was saying at the beginning. You have to preside over change and explain it – you've got to explain what you are doing and why.

You have to preside over change and explain it – you've got to explain what you are doing and why.

My advice to an incoming secretary of state is to know what you are doing, get stuck in and enjoy it. Health secretary was probably my biggest single challenge. The two jobs I've enjoyed most were health and the Treasury. I'm not sure which I enjoyed most, the Treasury probably, because you get into every form of government. But I enjoyed health. It was the toughest job I ever had, much tougher than the others.

The next secretary of state might have a calmer time because at the moment everybody has agreed on the diagnosis – not the public, but everybody else. It's the huge surge in the elderly with chronic conditions that has to be coped with, and what is badly wrong is that the tie-up between the hospital service, general practice and community care isn't working. Probably the next secretary of state will spend his time allowing NHS England to develop their plans, and assuming they don't make a mess of it, fighting off every pressure to start politicising it again.

'Chequers was surrounded by furious journalists and it was all hopeless.'

William Waldegrave
November 1990 – April 1992

Lord Waldegrave of North Hill was Secretary of State for Health from November 1990 to April 1992. He was also, at Cabinet level, Chief Secretary to the Treasury and Minister of Agriculture Fisheries and Food, while holding one ministerial position or another continuously from 1981 to 1997.

The job of the Secretary of State for Health depends on whether you think that the system, at any given time, is in need of policy reform.

I came to think it did. When I was appointed, Mrs T [Thatcher] said to me, 'Kenneth [Clarke] has stirred them all up, I want you to calm them all down again,' and then made it absolutely clear to me that if I wanted to just cut the throat of all these reforms that was fine as far as she was concerned. I then went along with Duncan Nichol and we had a meeting with her in Number 10, just before she went to Paris, just before she fell.

We persuaded her, and it was a matter of persuasion, that the thing made sense and wasn't just Kenneth trying to cause trouble. But it was clear that she had no particular commitment to it at all.

I became convinced that the idea of separating commissioning from provision was correct – the fundamental structure. Although I never could quite see where GP fundholders fitted in, except that they were a source of innovation in a rather random way round the place. And then there was a great to-do that we should have a pilot study somewhere.

I came under some pressure from the American guru, Alain Enthoven.* I respected him and I was partly converted by him. He pushed that it should be trialled somewhere and I said, 'You can't do a trial, the boundary conditions would be hopeless, and it wouldn't work at all. Nobody would be committed to it and the trial would certainly fail and what would happen on the boundaries' and so on. He wrote to me, incidentally, later on, saying I was quite right about that.

So back to the question of the role. There seemed to me to be a role there of trying to reform a system. It was one of the moments, rather like the moment in 1974, the end of Ted's [Heath] time, when they'd set up the regional health authorities. There was a real argument. Quintin Hogg [Lord Hailsham] argued in cabinet that they should be democratically elected, and we were doing local government reform at the same time. So, it was a watershed moment like that, in that there was a legitimate policy argument.

Is it possible, in any business or in any organisation, truly to separate policy from execution?

I then set up a policy board, or maybe what I did was refresh the policy board that Ken had set up. [The NHS Policy Board sat above the then NHS Management Board.] But then, the inherent difficulty of trying to separate the management from policy came back. I didn't want anybody else, perhaps wrongly, to be chairman of the policy board. So I made myself the chairman of it. It was implicitly saying that the secretary of state should not just be policy, but

---

* Alain Enthoven's Nuffield Trust paper *Reflections on the management of the National Health Service* Occasional Paper no 5, 1985, had provided much of the inspiration for the purchaser/provider split of the 1991 reforms.

should also be an executive. Perhaps I shouldn't have chaired it. But then this is the inherent difficulty of the whole thing – is it possible, in any business or in any organisation, truly to separate policy from execution?

I certainly thought then that to see the policy through, I had to retain the strategic control of what was happening with some kind of non-party political support, although doing anything was inherently political and Duncan Nichol [the NHS chief executive] was under political attack as well as management attack.

I saw the board's role to be overseeing of the establishment of the policy, of the structures. This was, of course, the grave difficulty. We had a great seminar at Chequers all about it just as the first trusts were being established. And the first thing that happened in one of the first trusts to be established – Guy's – was that a lot of nurses were fired.

And so Chequers was surrounded by furious journalists and it was all hopeless. One could see that actually, the famous and hopeless Aneurin Bevan remark about the bedpans and all that was always going to be true – which is fundamentally what's wrong with the system.

The policy board didn't do all that much. But I think it was a way of saying that there was something that the secretary of state had to do, which wasn't just saying, 'we've passed this Act of Parliament', but also saying that 'we have to see that the outcome bears some relationship to what we've done'.

It had some reasonably independent people on it. And I think it did some good in the early days, because we were going very fast. You always are in politics. You can't stop and say, 'We're going to wait and see what happens for a bit'. But its role was never thoroughly satisfactory. And the management of the information was very weak, and remains so I suspect.

Secretary of State for Health is the most powerful managerial job in Whitehall, or was then. If you were a powerful enough minister with enough coherence and enough support from senior management, you could actually change things. Even the Secretary of State for Defence can't do that. The chiefs of staff can just say 'no' and go to the prime minister if they want to. The job at work and pensions [where there are tens of thousands of staff delivering benefits] might be comparable, but I never did that one. And when health was part of the Department of Health and Social Security it does make one admire Norman Fowler and people like that who did both jobs in one – without ever breaking sweat as far as I can see. But health was completely different from any of the things I was used to, as in the Department of the Environment or the Department of Education.

It was by far the biggest secretary of state job that I had. I think chief secretary is quite important. But that is a completely different kind of job. It's like being a finance director of an enormous thing, going over everybody's plans, and negotiating with them, and trying to figure when they're lying and when they're not about what they need, and so on.

But, otherwise, I was minister of agriculture [a Cabinet post at the time]. Well, we don't have an agricultural policy in this country, because it's all the occupied field of the European Union. Being minister of agriculture was a European negotiating job, and we were always in the minority. I should think being minister of defence is a very big job. I would have liked to have done it.

Of course, they've made education rather like this [health] now. They think they're going to be able to run all the schools, those direct grant schools, from Whitehall, which is obviously completely bonkers and it will all end in tears. Well, it'll end up with regional organisations and then somebody will say, 'Well, we don't like these regional organisations.' Then we're back where we started. So, I mean, I have absolutely no certainty in my mind about how those things should be managed.

Here we are now dismantling these tiddly little banks like RBS and HSBC, which are tiny compared to the National

Health Service and everyone's completely agreed that you can't possibly manage a thing that has 66,000 employees like RBS. It's far too big, completely unmanageable; you need to break it up at once. And, here we are with the NHS. It's quite interesting.

But I didn't see the NHS as one organisation – it's made of hundreds of organisations. But it felt like that when the unions turned up – the BMA [British Medical Association] or NUPE [National Union of Public Employees, later merged into Unison] or COHSE [Confederation of Health Service Employees, likewise merged into Unison]. They were, of course, inherently centralising, by definition. They are organisations that wouldn't exist without a centralised thing to negotiate with. There were certainly very powerful centripetal forces. That was a centralised element, and one that it was odd that the secretary of state did – those bloody negotiations. The thing that subtracted more years of my life than practically anything else was doing the dentists' negotiation.

I didn't see the NHS as one organisation – it's made of hundreds of organisations.

What a secretary of state was doing negotiating with these dentists – they always out-manoeuvred us. There should have been somebody else doing it. That was a hopeless way of doing procurement, which is what it was. It's like sending the secretary of defence to negotiate with Lockheed. Perhaps they do and perhaps that's why that's always over the top too. But the unions are always, of course, very skilful at saying, 'We must meet the minister'.

And anything where the minister is standing, ultimately, in front of the House of Commons and taking the blame for everything is hugely upwardly centralising. And if you're to blame for some frightful situation that somebody in Staffordshire has made, then you feel you have to have levers to be able to protect yourself. But, I think, maybe, we've got better at that. I don't see the secretary of state being held wholly personally accountable for local catastrophes now, in quite the same way. You see them being held accountable for what response the system produces. But that's better, that's an improvement. In my day, if Mid Staffs had occurred, the secretary of state would have had to visit there and it would have been a nightmare. That has been slowly changing, for the better.

Except that you then have the question of, 'What about the accountability of the boards of the trusts?' and, 'What about the accountability of the boards of the commissioners?' and how does that work? We used to draw diagrams [back at the time of the 1991 reforms]. The logical line of accountability was all through the commissioning side. The democratic system set the priorities in consultation, you'd hope, with local interests. Those were reflected through commissioning. And then the commissioners tried to find the best provision to meet the need. It all made a certain beautiful, logical sense.

The logical line of accountability was all through the commissioning side.

You shouldn't be, as the secretary of state, accountable at all for the providers, except that, for reasons of history, the great majority of the providers belonged to the state. So, you had to be at least accountable for them not stealing the money, and audit and propriety and so on. The theory was that the minister should do the prioritising, but not run the services. Do we need more money on sickle cell anaemia, or old age? But that was based on a theory – on the Alain Enthoven-like theory, if you like – that all the hospitals belonged to someone else. To charities or businesses or something, for which you did not have direct responsibility.

Did I feel I had command and control? Well, in the sense that if I'd given an order to do something, if I'd said, 'We are going to close Frenchay Hospital and move it to somewhere else,' and persuaded people to do X and Y, one could probably have done that. But if command and control means did I feel that I was in control of what was going on in Frenchay Hospital? No. Not at all.

Of course one's other job was to get enough money for the NHS. I was in a strong position, because we were coming up to an election [1992]. So I got lots of money and they squirreled it away for several years afterwards.

Another example of the improvement is that we had a tremendous row about some cancer drug that was or wasn't available. The systems set up now mean that nobody seems to worry the health secretary about that. They argue with NICE and so on and that's much more rational. Although the prime minister, slightly dangerously, intervened with the Cancer Drugs Fund.

NICE was a very good thing and there was a proto-NICE, which I did have something to do with, beginning to be set up. But the concept of trying to have some rational cost-benefit analysis and not just have whatever the *Daily Mail* thought the money should be spent on must be right. I think NICE is one of the best innovations.

I'm also intrigued by what is happening in Manchester. I do think there's a powerful logic, even if you keep the means testing, for putting the health and social care as one ring-fenced budget.

That was always passionately opposed by the Treasury, because the Treasury's nightmare was always that you would push the frontier out and then the whole thing would be non-means tested and we'd be paying for a full health and social care system. That certainly won't happen unless we're very, very rich, or feeling very, very rich.

And although health is ring-fenced, the social care part won't be in the Manchester scheme. That will end in tears, I suspect. But even so I am very excited by the Manchester approach.

I suppose what I'm implicitly saying by all this is that the right policy change is to get to a situation where the framework for policy and the expenditure of state money is obviously for the minister to negotiate with his colleagues. But, that if you've got a sensible framework, managerially, then he should not be involved much managerially.

He or she is bound to have to appoint the very senior people, so they are going to be accountable for who they have appointed. But they should try and stand back from it. I'm not up to date enough to comment sensibly on the statutorily independent board that Lansley set up.

But whether it really is a single managerial job under any model, you're certainly not going to find a politician who's trained to do that. But then, the theory of fragmentation, of the providers, in particular, was that nobody can manage a thing bigger than a big hospital trust and that's difficult enough to manage.

Perhaps there's no perfect model. What happens in France, or somewhere like that? The grass is always greener and all that kind of thing. There have been huge strikes over pay in France. I remember them turning the fire hoses on the nurses in my day. Which we wouldn't have got away with.

There was never a moment when one didn't think one was wrestling with real problems and that this was what public service was about.

It was the most demanding job I had. On a good day it was satisfying, but I had an election looming over me the whole period, and I'm not the greatest electioneer and I didn't much care for any of that. But it was hugely satisfying in that there was never a moment when one didn't think one was wrestling with real problems and that this was what public service was about.

And very satisfying in that you dealt with a good section of the smartest and most impressive people in the whole country, at the top of the various pyramids and the bottom of the various pyramids. But, there was the constantly looming feeling that you would wake up in the morning and there would be some frightful thing in the paper and that you were in trouble. The slightly cheerful press officer ringing you at 5:30 in the morning saying, 'I'm terribly sorry to wake you secretary of state, but there's a rather unfortunate story', and so on. The pressure of it is very, very great. You have to be as tough as old boots, like Ken, to relish it all.

So it's satisfying, but high risk, and you certainly don't want to do it if you can, as a Tory minister, in the run-up to an election. Although, then you don't get any money, probably, if you're not in the run-up to an election. And I could get the money.

'Sometimes you want a window breaker and sometimes you want a glazier.'

Virginia Bottomley
April 1992 – July 1995

Baroness Bottomley of Nettlestone was Minister of State for Health from October 1989 to April 1992 and Secretary of State for Health from April 1992 to July 1995. She was also Minister of State at the Department of the Environment and Secretary of State for National Heritage.

I think I was in some ways quite different to others and because I brought three key principles that I understood to the party. The first was that I understood what leadership was about and big organisations need leaders. Whatever way you look at it, politicians aren't leaders. They don't understand about the long term. They're not with you for the thick and thin. They suddenly move at the toss of a hat. I would have liked to have been that long-term leader, but I knew I couldn't be.

I knew the leader was the chief executive. And I was very fortunate. I had a very high regard for Duncan Nichol and a very high regard for Alan Langlands [successive chief executives of the NHS]. I knew that if you really want people to do difficult things on a Friday night when the A&E is imploding, they don't do it because they have politicians issuing hyperbole; they do it for their leaders. And the leader is not a politician. It is the chief executive or the leader of their trust.

So my great theme was how could you help them be leaders? So that you really empower the organisation? I completely understood that they needed leadership, but at the same time I felt, as secretary of state in the health service, I didn't want – my great quip was – 'I don't want them to hear the hospital is closing from the NUPE official on News at Ten.' [National Union of Public Employees, later merged into Unison].

I really wanted to have a proper communication system that came through from the secretary of state, through the system. I got very distressed about leaks and for that reason I was most unsuitable for a 21st century politician – because I didn't believe in leaks myself because I felt you should communicate down the line. This is an extraordinarily old-fashioned approach.

Second, I was very influenced by Keith Joseph, and Keith Joseph always used to refer to the 'holder of my office'. And what he meant by that was that being a secretary of state is a custodianship. It's a guardianship. I was a magistrate when I was very young. I was 27, and I was chairman of the juvenile court when I was 32. When you were chairman of the court, you were the holder of the office. It wasn't Virginia Bottomley. I felt that very strongly in the office of secretary of state. This was a custodianship. It was funded by the taxpayer. I wasn't there because I was Labour or Tory or Liberal. So I had this very strong sense of propriety about how to behave and how to discharge the role, and this sense of stewardship. I realise that most people just don't think in those terms.

The third thing that influenced me deeply was when Margaret Thatcher made me a minister. I was absolutely flabbergasted, because I knew Mrs Thatcher didn't really approve of me. I said, 'I don't know anything about it' – because this was going into the Department of the Environment. And she said, 'Well, in that case we'll have to read it up.' Of course all politicians, all men in particular say, 'Well prime minister, I will bring a clear mind to the problem.' They just never say, 'I don't know anything about it…'

But the one thing she said, which always stuck in my mind, is 'never turn down the opportunity to explain the government's case, because nobody else will'. The other thing I felt, this is an organisation that's got a million people, there are patients, users who are all very emotional and 'no comment' isn't good enough. The message needs to be communicated. Now alongside my view that the NHS leaders should lead, at that time they

'never turn down the opportunity to explain the government's case, because nobody else will.'

were extremely reluctant to communicate in any way at all in the public domain. I think these days the local NHS people are much more likely to speak up. So I used to get very exercised about that. The story on the six o'clock news on the Today programme. And if the story is distorted at six, it's a sort of herd of elephants running down not only Whitehall – which did worry me a little bit – but I was always more concerned about the anxiety it provoked in people throughout the health service. That they all think that this is going to happen or that is going to happen and nobody is giving them the reasons. So I felt really strongly that it should be addressed.

So I was on the phone to the press officer, or the chief medical officer, or whoever, to get it addressed. And the other thing, which is so much me, is what I learnt from Nick Ridley [Secretary of State for the Environment when Bottomley was minister of state]. His view was that if it is good news you give it to the parliamentary secretary to announce. If it is bad news, the secretary of state does it. It's all about my great uncles walking towards the guns, a sort of stoicism that as a leader you had to do the heavy lifting and walk toward the guns. The difficult things, like Beverley Allitt [the nurse convicted of murdering four children and attempting to murder three more on an NHS ward]… I needed to take responsibility for difficult news. I can't imagine how I survived at all!

The result of all this was I had an extraordinary good relationship with the civil servants and the people I worked with. I think the politicians mostly thought I wasn't much use. But the people I worked with who were doing the heavy lifting, it was very harmonious and a lot of trust and mutual respect.

So my role was to make sure we tackled the problems that weren't going to go away. So there had already been 29 reports into London hospitals. It needed action, not options. So my stoical personality said, 'Right, we must do this.' So we had the big London hospitals' reorganisation and the decision to close Barts and the enormous rows that went with all of that.

We had these top of the office meetings every Wednesday with the permanent secretary, the chief executive of the NHS, the chief medical officer and the head of social services, an arrangement I think I inherited from William [Waldegrave]. I always called everybody rather formally by their title, because it was a reminder of what they're there for. And I had some sharp words with Richard Wilson, the cabinet secretary, when Alan Milburn merged the post of permanent secretary and NHS chief executive. I said, 'You must have a permanent secretary. The permanent secretary deals with endless turf wars, honours, dodgy special advisers, incoming health ministers – the department needs a permanent secretary.' I think when Labour came in they lost, or didn't understand, the formality of the structure. I knew how the different components worked.

In my time, we had the regional chairmen. I had a lot of time for them. They were very important. I was always very careful not just to appoint Conservatives because I remember when David Ennals came in [Labour Secretary of State for Social Services, 1976–1979] they sacked more than 100 Tory chairmen. So you lose continuity and you lose knowledge, and it's almost another reorganisation. And I said to John Major, 'we've just got to appoint the best people, regardless of party. It's our NHS, not the Tories' NHS.' The NHS was very tribal, so you had nurses, doctors, managers. You could feel them getting in their bunkers. And the regional chairmen could knock heads together. Handle disputes and tensions, all those sort of things. And they were people to whom MPs of all parties could go with their concerns and problems about the NHS.

How far can you take the politics out? Well Ken [Clarke] set up the NHS Executive in Leeds to try to get that sort of separation. That involved an awful lot of first-class tickets, and chat on trains! Ken absolutely believed in principle that the executive and the trusts should be more autonomous. He absolutely believed that politicians should be away from the direct management. My instincts were more to worry away, if there was a problem, know what the problem was. The old bedpan metaphor continues to run.

My instincts were more to worry away, if there was a problem, know what the problem was.

And there was an NHS Policy Board of outside advisers which he'd also set up. I'd have regular meetings with the regional chairmen every two months, and then there was the policy board, which might have been very useful when the NHS reforms were being set up. But creating agendas for both became ridiculous. You tell me Stephen Dorrell abolished it. Well, he was completely right.

My advice for incoming ministers? If you want to keep this Herculean project working, you've got to trouble it with as few petty initiatives as possible. Every minister needs their own pet project – pink sheets for girls, blue sheets for boys, get you seen in a fortnight, whatever. Tempting as it is, this is a total diversion of energy. I had a dinner once for leaders from different industries. The NHS person said he had 120 targets. The person from BAE had three targets. There are some basic lessons people should learn about how you run a business, how you motivate people. A lot of people now really know nothing about managing and leading organisations because politicians increasingly are one-man bands, because of their background. Alan Johnson had run a trade union, and he was very good because he knew how to create a coalition.

This is a connected thought. But it's quite fun. The great thing about Roy Griffiths [who undertook the NHS Management Inquiry] was that he was company secretary and much else at Sainsbury's, when it was a family firm. And when you have a family firm you have to find a job for the clever one, the financial one, the marketing one, the stupid one. Ministers are like that. Ministers are not like a normal business where they're handpicked for their competence. They're picked for all sorts of reasons. So you had one from the north, one from the south, one from a trade union background, one for this, that and the other. Then you have to find roles for them, which will play to their strengths.

I came to like the idea of an NHS chairman and a more independent board. Or some distance from ministers for the NHS. So the parallel is that the Ministry of Defence used to have a chief of the defence staff, or the Bank of England has the governor, who is over and beyond party politics. You should get as close to that as you can. But there are different times in politics, and it does go in cycles. Sometimes you want a window breaker and sometimes you want a glazier. Ken was a window breaker and he was brilliant. But after that you get William Waldegrave who was a glazier. And my job, after the election [in 1992], was that we'd got some trusts and fundholders up and running and my task was to get all of that beyond a tipping point. Quieten it all down. Show them you care. And then a new set of problems will arrive and you need a Ken to break the windows again.

'Of course it doesn't work if you change it every five years.'

Stephen Dorrell
July 1995 – May 1997

Rt Hon Stephen Dorrell was Minister of State for Health from 1990 to 1992 and Secretary of State for Health from July 1995 to May 1997. He was also Secretary of State for National Heritage.

The role of the Secretary of State for Health is determined to some extent by the views and the attitudes of the incumbent. Secondly, by the attitudes and views of the prime minister of the day. And thirdly, and mostly importantly, by the attitudes of the voters.

The right order actually is to put the voters first, the incumbent second and the prime minister third, probably. Because it is not much [good] you going to the voters and saying, 'I'm not responsible for this.' The obvious response from them is, 'If you can't do anything about it, what use are you?' So, the voter thinks that the health secretary is responsible if something goes wrong and the health secretary should be held accountable. And that's the starting point.

Then you come to the question of the attitudes of the incumbent. I have a very strong view about what the role ought to be and how you ought to discharge it – which is that you're not responsible for making all the decisions, and it's the old,

I suspect misquoted thing about the bedpan in South Wales. What you are responsible for is outcomes and structures and incentives. You are responsible for the effect of the decisions, but you're not responsible for the decisions themselves.

To take it beyond the level of generality. In the Lincolnshire health economy, for example, if there isn't joined up health and social care then somebody will ask the health secretary why that isn't the case, and what are they going to do about it? Now, that doesn't mean the health secretary gets on a train to Lincoln to do it. But it does mean that if the system doesn't work then they're held to account for the fact that it doesn't work.

There is nothing unique to the health service about this. It's true in any large organisation, that the chief executive who tries to make every decision quickly finds that they're lost. Well run organisations invest a considerable amount of time and effort in insisting that decisions are taken as close as possible to the point where the information is good.

First of all you haven't got the bandwidth. You can't do everything at the centre. But secondly, however good the information is at the centre it is always less good than at the front line. So empowered local management is bound to be better informed. That does not always mean it makes a good decision. But it is bound to be better informed, and therefore is better placed to make good decisions than people further up the line. But the secretary of state is responsible for the outcome of those decisions, notably when it goes wrong, because when it goes right people remember it afterwards with a vague warm glow. If you come into politics looking for bouquets you're in the wrong line of country.

However good the information is at the centre it is always less good than at the front line.

And then there is the view of the prime minister, and real life, in the run-up to an election in particular. I guess that for the prime minister the health secretary is a kind of risk manager.

I often say that the prime minister of any party is party blind. They only have one objective for a health secretary, which is to keep the NHS out of the newspapers – because if it's in the newspapers it's for the reason we just touched on. It's always there for bad reasons not good, or almost always. So the incumbent of Richmond House, from the prime minister's perspective, is the person responsible for keeping the health service out of the newspapers – risk management. That's what leads health secretaries into what I think is a blind alley, which is believing that risk management is best delivered by more control. But control and intervention disempowers management in any organisation. Again, this is a universal truth. It's true in textiles, it's true in engineering, and it's true in health care. The more you intervene, the less effective management is, and therefore the higher the risk that you're allegedly trying to manage.

So yes, as you put it, I did try to behave like chairman of the board, not chief executive of the National Health Service. But when people said to me what did I think about the coalition setting up an independent board, I used to say, 'Well I am the person who abolished the last one!'

It wasn't independent and it made no pretence to be. But there was a policy board which Ken Clarke had set up. So there were these two big regular meetings in the Cathedral Room at Richmond House. One was the regional chairmen, which did have some purpose. The other was the Policy Board. There were these various panjandrums from the world of business and elsewhere, who were going to tell the Department of Health how to run a multibillion-pound corporation.

I remember going to these things when Ken was secretary of state and not really getting it. But then, I was a junior minister so I just went along with it. I think I cancelled two or maybe even three meetings of this assembly at short notice, thinking I had better ways of spending my time, and it became an embarrassment. It had got to point where it either had to meet or I had to abolish it. So I abolished it.

As you know I voted for the 2012 Act and there were reasons why I did so, and I am quite happy to defend why I voted for it. But all this stuff about creating independent decision making and getting the health service out of politics blah, blah, blah… Well, that's exactly the same speech that we used to make in favour of the health authorities that were statutorily independent. They existed in statute. They had responsibilities defined in statute. So what's changed?

I've never quite believed these parallels with the BBC or the Bank of England's independence. The BBC is completely different. Voters don't need to be persuaded that journalism should be independent of politics. They don't want politicians interfering, so that one's easy to explain. The Bank of England is trickier. But essentially it only has one target, which is much easier than the NHS which is full of competing desirable outcomes. I was an advocate of an independent Bank. But we don't yet know, in truth, how the voters will react if inflation gets out of control because the Bank has got its interest rate policy seriously wrong. When we get to that, then we'll know how well the voters take to the principle of an independent Bank of England. Will they really accept that Mark Carney has an existence in their lives independent of George Osborne when Mark Carney or his successor bogs up and George says it's nothing to do with him? That will be the test.

As far as voters are concerned, the ministers were responsible for the reconfiguration that they'd allowed to happen. You can't legislate away responsibility.

You make the point that the Independent Reconfiguration Panel has helped. Yes, okay. But I don't think there are many voters, to go back to that test, who have ever heard of the Independent Reconfiguration Panel. I think that it's helped – because within the political class it's given one politician an excuse to make to another politician. But it's all an insiders' game, and it reflects the will of ministers at that time –

to allow a process to take place and to give themselves excuses. I think that's all insider talk. As far as voters are concerned, the ministers were responsible for the reconfiguration that they'd allowed to happen. You can't legislate away responsibility.

You've heard me say it, times without number, that actually health policy hasn't changed. Frank Dobson would like to have changed it and wasn't able to. But apart from him, no health secretary has wanted to change policy since 1991, which is the day when it really did change. We used to have a provider-led system; we now have a commissioner-led system. That is different, but it's the last time anybody fundamentally changed health policy. The question lies between the concept and the execution. That's where the story is – and the disability, the powerlessness of commissioners, is the result of consistent execution failure. But that's hardly surprising when successive governments have reorganised the commissioner side every five years. Well, of course it doesn't work if you change it every five years.

Incidentally, of course, it doesn't work if you have NHS England commissioning primary care, NHS England doing specialist care, 'clinical commissioning groups land', 'social service land' and so on – and if you really want to make it sound complicated you can introduce various other elements. The whole health landscape is impenetrably complicated.

It was somewhat clearer in the days when we had health authorities. But we've never had primary and secondary commissioning together, and we've never really had joined-up commissioning between health and social care, or social housing.

Which is why I'm in favour of health and wellbeing boards. It's one of the things I agree with Andy Burnham about. As you've heard me say, I agree – or more precisely, he agrees with me, because we voted for it first – that these are potentially catalysts to bring together a simple commissioning process. It's the old principle of KISS, 'Keep It Simple, Stupid'.

My advice to an incoming health secretary is stick to the policy that all health secretaries except Frank have pursued – of developing commissioning. In the end, the health secretary is the commissioner in chief. So actually, they should stop obsessing about hospital management, which is anyway a fraction of care delivery. Recognise you are commissioner in chief, accept responsibility for the commissioning process, and make it work.

Stop obsessing about hospital management, which is anyway a fraction of care delivery.

I'm sceptical about an independent board. If it all goes pear-shaped, will the voters hold Simon Stevens to account? Of course they won't. You've heard me say it before, but I think we fought a civil war on this principle in the 1640s, and as I remember, the principle of accountability won!

You are right that policy and implementation are intertwined. One of the reasons I enjoyed the health ministerial roles is that in our system health politics is actually a unique combination of public policy, social policy and management. There is lots and lots of policy around the place, and every minister has some degree of management exposure. But no other minister is responsible for management decisions on the scale that the health secretary is. What do the voters want? They want equitable access, which is policy, to high quality health care, which is pure operations. So, within half a dozen or so words which summarise the mission of the health service, 'equitable access to high quality health care', you've got operations and strategy all mixed up in a single short sentence. The health secretary's job is unique in that there is a largely nationalised supply sector. It is by far the largest nationalised industry, and the health secretary is, as a matter of fact, responsible for it.

That still means you work to get decisions taken as close as possible to where the information is good. The moment you insist on taking a decision at the centre that is properly in the scope of one of the people that you employ, you've disabled management. That's basic management theory. It's all about pushing it down. If you don't do that, you have a bunch of disempowered managers. And at the moment I think there is a big shift to the centre, and I think that's very dangerous. People in foundation trusts who thought trust status put things in their scope of responsibility are now being asked to fill in forms and account for it up the line, and beyond that to the political world. Personally, I think that is a big mistake.

'I have no problems with command and control.'

Frank Dobson
May 1997 – October 1999

Rt Hon Frank Dobson was Secretary of State for Health from May 1997 to October 1999.

I think the secretary of state has two roles. One is to implement all reasonable things which were included in the election manifesto as keeping election promises is a most important part of politics. The failure to do so is the most damaging part. The second is to try to help all the people involved do their jobs as well as they would like to do them, by removing obstructions and lunacies out of their way and really trying to make the system work, rather than constantly tinkering and pissing around with it. Which was an alien concept as far as the Blairite Downing Street was concerned, who wanted an initiative every 20 minutes.

There is an important role for ministers. Because there isn't really this distinction that people like to make between policy and management. Take NHS Direct for example, which we set up.

The civil servants came to me and said we've got this idea for a nurse-led helpline. And there were three computer protocols or algorithms for them to use to triage the patients. I asked them how they were going to choose between them, and they said 'from our experience' and they wanted to introduce it nationwide – 'bam' – all on one day. And I said how long is this going to take? And they said 18 months.

Well, thinking both backwards at the time, and, as it turns out, forward, everything that central government has ever done to do with a computer nationwide has been a fuck up, without fail. So I said: 'No. We're going to take three years. And we will have three pilots of each of these algorithms, and then gradually spread it.' And the British protocol turned out to be bloody useless.

Then there was a young man called Jenkins who was in charge of it. And this is an oddity of the importance of ministers as well. Every deadline was being met. Every standard was being met. And it was gradually being spread across the country. Then I heard, entirely by accident, Jenkins had been moved. So I said to the perm sec, 'What's going on?' He said, 'Well it is career development.' So I said, 'But this isn't the Ministry of Career Development, it's the Ministry of Health and Social Services. Get him back.'

It wouldn't have happened without me just saying, 'That's what I want, go off and do it.' And that is management really.

'But he's been promoted, he's getting extra money.' 'So he should be promoted,' I said, 'and given extra money. Get him back.' And he was, I understand, very happy to come back and it was all duly implemented. So that was, I think, an example of important ministerial involvement. It wouldn't have happened without me just saying, 'That's what I want, go off and do it.' And that is management really.

It may have helped that before I was an MP I worked for the Central Electricity Generating Board and I had to organise things and get them done. I worked at making things work before I was an MP. So that may have coloured my view.

Take meningitis C, for which there was a new vaccine. We all knew it was killing about 100 toddlers a year and maiming about another 1,000 for life. And first of all I was told there was no money for a new vaccine. Nothing in the budget. So I said: 'Gordon Brown is paying out billions to fucking farmers to compensate them for killing cattle with CJD [Creutzfeldt-Jakob disease] and you are suggesting we can't find the money!' So we found the money. And then there wasn't enough vaccine to do everyone, and officialdom wanted to wait until there was. So I said: 'So we are going to hold it back while toddlers are dying, being maimed for life, are we?'… 'Well now you put it like that…'

And I collaborated throughout with David Salisbury who was the chairman of the Joint Committee on Vaccination and Immunisation, who was livid about the attitude of the machine towards it. So there was clearly not going to be enough vaccine for all the toddlers and the people I refer to as the snoggers – the people who were going to college for the first time.

So we ended up with a formula which was that the littlies would get the new one straight away and there would be a big drive to get the snoggers to get the existing meningitis C vaccine, which had the disadvantage that its effectiveness hung on in the body for about two to three years, whereas the new one was lifelong or something or like that.

Wyeth say they can't produce enough, even for that set of priorities. And the boss comes over from the States to see me. And should I shout at him, or say, 'We've got a problem, the pair of us.' I did the latter because shouting has never got me to do anything, so I don't think it does very many other people.

He goes away and they come back saying, 'I am sorry we can only produce about half of what you need.' 'Bugger.' Then David Salisbury comes loping in, and he did lope, comes in about 10 days later and says, 'Oh it's all right. There is a small chemical company in Switzerland who is brewing it up and they had a contract to somebody else and Wyeth have bought out the other contract. So they can do it.'

It was all developed with the meningitis charities and with the British Medical Association whose GP chairman, John Chisholm, was incredibly helpful. I am sitting having breakfast and on the Today programme on the first day it starts, this bloke comes on, going on about, 'It's all a disaster I can't get the vaccine that I need, etc, etc…' I am absolutely livid and about 10 minutes later, unprompted by me or anybody in the department, John Chisholm fought his way on to the Today programme and said, 'This bloke must be blind because if he turned over the page of the paper he was quoting from it gave him about four telephone numbers where he could get it sorted out. This has been a brilliant collaborative effort by everybody, so piss off.'

It was the only thing favourable to the NHS that there has ever been on the Today programme as far as I know. So that was ministerial involvement as well, as was how we dealt with CJD and blood.

I believe Simon Stevens once referred to me as wandering up and down the ministerial corridor in my stockinged feet, like the non-executive chairman who knew what he was doing. I took that as a compliment really.

So my attitude to policy was, 'Okay, right that's the policy, well how do we implement it?' Because there isn't a Rolls Royce machine that is going to implement it. At the very last cabinet meeting I went to, before I foolishly resigned [to run as London mayor], there was a discussion about the civil service and everyone was saying 'oh, it's perfect' and I said 'well I don't think it is perfect. It is not the fault of the top civil servants because they are displaying the characteristics of what has been expected of them. But it tends to be staffed by people who produce a learned treaty on why the latest initiative has failed, rather than getting somebody who from the start makes sure it works.' And suddenly everyone was saying 'oh, but you are absolutely right'.

So my attitude to policy was, 'Okay, right that's the policy, well how do we implement it?'

I exclude Alan Langlands from that. And Herbert Laming [Chief Inspector of Social Services]. I had a very, very high opinion of Alan Langlands. But it was the departmental civil servants, plus the impact of the Treasury and of Downing Street. One of the things that is ignored in a lot of these analyses of processes within government is that there is a lot of attention paid to the political appointees in Downing Street. But it is chock full of civil servants, and civil servants in departments who don't want to do something get in touch with the civil servants in Downing Street to try to get Downing Street to come back crashing down on the minister, to stop the minister forcing through the minister's policies. There is a sort of triangular relationship.

The other oddity was that when I arrived, the PM wants to see us. 'Us' was me, the perm sec and Alan Langlands. So I said, 'Why not Ken Calman – the chief medical officer?' All three of Langlands, the perm sec and the CMO are permanent secretary grade. And they said: 'Oh well, Ken Calman doesn't get involved in policy things and such like.' I said, 'Well he does now.' So I used to insist that he went with us. It may have been a personality thing, but the idea that major issues are going to be discussed with the prime minister and the chief medical officer isn't going to be there, seemed to me quite bizarre.

You put it to me that my period was seen as a period of strong command and control because there were a lot of centrally decided initiatives – setting up NICE, and the Commission for Health Improvement, National Service Frameworks, spending money on NHS Direct and Walk-In Centres and refurbishing A&E departments and cutting waiting lists – so people tend to see it as a period of quite strong command and control, because there were very clear decisions on what the available cash was to be spent on. Well, I entirely agree with that. I have no problems with command and control. It is part of the secretary of state's job.

Take prostheses for example. We were still giving people wooden legs! And hearings aids. A standard NHS hearing aid cost £60, and 50% of them whistled and bleeped so badly that half the people put them in a drawer after about a fortnight. So that was £60 spent on something that was useless. At that time the new electronic ones were about £1,000. So I say: 'Well supposing we offer to buy a job lot of half a million, or a quarter of a million, or whatever it was?' They came down to about £120. So my view then was, 'Well £120 on something that works is a better bargain than £60 on something that doesn't.' So there were things like that which I did.

As for the current split of NHS England as a statutorily independent commissioning board? Well it is bollocks. Take an example of something much cruder – the Potters Bar train crash. The railways were denationalised but it wasn't the privately owned operators who appeared at the despatch box to answer for it. It was the minister of transport who got a kicking over it, and people would be more likely to accept some sort of non-responsibility on the railways compared with the NHS. The idea therefore that the NHS is going to be this independent organisation, without political interference, and this, that and the other, is just rubbish and it has proved to be just rubbish.

Every time anything crops up the secretary of state intervenes and blames somebody else. Because this distancing has meant that he can blame somebody else but not accept any blame himself. Which I think was probably the object of the exercise. But it doesn't mean that there isn't political interference.

In law he doesn't have this direct responsibility. But nobody believes it really, and he clearly is interfering all the time. What is noticeable of course is that when anything goes wrong it is not a minister who goes on the telly and radio anymore, it is one of the officials – trying to justify 111 for instance and things like that.

I think the person who takes the decisions should carry the can and the person who carries the can should take the decisions. There isn't any way in the end, in this country for the next 25 years, even if the present dispensation remained in place, that people will not expect the health secretary to be responsible, and take the blame when things go wrong.

My advice to an incoming Secretary of State for Health? Well, I was much criticised because I said to some reporter from the *Daily Mirror* who came to see me that the first thing I was going to do was sit down and have a good think! Which is out of fashion really isn't it, to sit down and have a good think? I think they need to do that.

Have a good think. And clearly there needs to be a better arrangement between the hospital services, GPs, health visitors, community services, social services, voluntary sector and God knows who. And there would be a real danger in saying we have got to have a universal approach that applies in Cumbria and Lewisham. So try a dozen pilot schemes on how best to do it and have a few pilot schemes in places where there is nobody with much enthusiasm for it. Because there is a danger if your pilot schemes are run by people who are enthusiastic and energetic they may make them work. And then you say to 25 other places, where that doesn't apply, 'Do what they have done.' And it won't work because there isn't the commitment, there isn't the energy, there isn't the thought put into it.

And what you have clearly got to do is to stop all this fragmentation. Because the idea that fragmented organisations entering into legally binding contracts with one another about the delivery of their bit of the service will produce a coordinated service is clearly totally loony.

Before we had this purchaser/provider split, the NHS spent four pence in the pound on administration, and it now spends at least 12. So that is £8bn more going on administration because of the money following the patient and all these bloody contracts and Christ knows what. So I think that the first thing the new health secretary should say is: 'Well let's try to cut back on all this crap.'

'Politics is the trap. And the only thing that can break it is politics.'

Alan Milburn
October 1999 – June 2003

Rt Hon Alan Milburn was Secretary of State for Health between October 1999 and June 2003. He was also Chief Secretary to the Treasury and Minister for the Cabinet Office. He was Minister of State for Health between 1997 and 1998.

I mean the job has clearly evolved and is evolving. It's actually easy to define in an organogram and really hard to do in practice. In an organogram you try to define it as successive secretaries of state from the different parties have sought to do, really from Ken Clarke onwards. You separate yourself from the operations, and deal with the strategic. That is the theory. The only thing that buggers it is the practice!

It is not a bad idea to start with the theory. The theory is you have a Secretary of State for Health, who is what it says on the tin – responsible for health in the broadest sense of the word. In our system, funded from general taxation, there's a custodian role to play and an accountability to discharge. So it is a perfectly sensible idea to have a Secretary of State for Health whose job primarily is about improving the health of the population and focusing upon how strategically the system as a whole should go about doing that.

Some people use metaphors of chief executive and chairman, but I don't think that is the right metaphor. I think it is much more a division of labour between setting overall objectives, aligning resources behind objectives, sticking to strategy, and keeping out of operations, broadly.

We've got to a very different model today. Organisationally and architecturally, it's a different model. But culturally and politically, it isn't. We changed some architecture but we haven't changed culture and we haven't changed politics. That's why it's really hard. Because every time there's a problem – guess what? Some poor bugger, whether it's me or Ken or Jeremy [Hunt], will get dragged to the despatch box and have to answer for themselves.

I'm afraid there is not a surfeit of politicians who think that their historical purpose, having got power, is somehow to give it away.

In the end, the only thing that can break that is politics. Politics is the trap. And the only thing that can break it is politics. I'm afraid there is not a surfeit of politicians who think that their historical purpose, having got power, is somehow to give it away. That's what you've got to do. That's what, in a sense, Ken was trying to do. That, in the end, with foundation trusts and markets and all that stuff, is what I was trying to do. That's an uncompleted journey.

One shouldn't be naïve about it, and simply assume that if only one had a strong enough personality type everything would be okay. Actually it's a real thing. People feel viscerally [about the accountability]. The public do, the media do. The NHS feels viscerally about it itself.

In that horrendous winter when I first became secretary of state, the press office was being flooded with questions from local newspapers about the terrible performance in Leeds, or Newcastle or Carlisle, you name it, wherever, and were answering the questions, until I stopped them doing so.

I basically said, 'Actually, it's not the job of you to answer a question about what's going on in Leeds.' It's the job of people in Leeds to answer that. It's possible to do it but you've got to design architecture that saves you from yourself.

So when Alan Johnson wanted to intervene in Mid Staffs, post my time, and found that he couldn't really do so, that was because intentionally I'd designed it in a way that it was impossible to do… well, not impossible, because he found a way to do it. Yes, of course.

So, as you say, behaviour trumps legislation. Absolutely it does. However, that isn't an argument against constructing architecture. It's an argument for constructing architecture but recognising that isn't enough. It's a necessary but not sufficient condition for change.

Have we constructed enough architecture that saves the secretary of state, whoever it is, from him or herself? No, we haven't. That's a journey that has still got to be completed.

The two really contentious things when we were writing the first white paper back in 1997 was not the primary care trusts and whatever but the Commission for Health Improvement, because that was going to bring an externality to the NHS, and NICE, the National Institute for Clinical Excellence.

The pharmaceutical industry was going to go mad, and GPs were going to go mad, because it would second guess both the market and referring decisions. None of that [in the long run] happened.

It's interesting to understand why NICE has been a successful and sustainable part of the architecture. I think some of the design features were good. It was constructed in a way that didn't purely separate it from politics. I don't know really how it works now, but in my day we would set the mandate, deciding what NICE would look at next. And I'd say to Mike Rawlins, 'Can you look at this bucket of cancer drugs?' or whatever. So it wasn't purely doing science. It was doing science at the behest of politics. We set the work programme in consultation with

NICE. But 'here's the steer, this is what we want you to look at – and it would be jolly nice if actually there were more yeses than nos.' I remember you [Nicholas Timmins] writing in the very early days, 'is NICE a force for rationing, or is it a force for expenditure?' It was a force for expenditure. You basically gave it a mandate to go and act, but you saved yourself from the position of making a decision, item by item, and indeed when the answer was 'no'. So it recognised the force of politics, and it got the right division of labour.

Second, it established a body of really credible science that almost made its case, in virtually every case, inarguable. What's so interesting is that despite the enormous resources of big pharma, by and large it hasn't won much against NICE, even in a very contentious or divisive decision. And third, it had continuity of personnel, which has actually been the most important thing – Andrew [Dillon, the Chief Executive] and Mike Rawlins [Chair between 1998 and 2013] – their double act and their personal credibility. In a funny sort of way that was both a problem and a protection for successive secretaries of state. There are design features you can replicate. It's not enough. So we've had the Cancer Drugs Fund. But at least that had to be an addendum to the architecture.

I think we are two-thirds of the way on the journey. So we had the purchaser/provider split, and then patient choice, and then the disaggregation of the system into independent, more autonomous organisations. And then the new regulatory architecture. I've got no idea what the Department of Health does any more because all those functions have either been disaggregated down or they've been disaggregated sideways. The really hard bit is you get the architecture and then you get Alan Johnson saying, 'fuck the system'. What do you do about that?

Let's presume that you could complete it, because broadly there is a political consensus, believe it or not. I mean one isn't going to hear much about that in the next few months [during the election campaign]. But broadly, Labour and Tory, in terms of architecture, are broadly on the same page. It's in no one's interest to say that but that's, I think, true. That's the easy bit.

…broadly, Labour and Tory, in terms of architecture, are broadly on the same page.

In a rational world, why would you want to be responsible for something over which one, you really have precious little locus or leverage, and two, why would you want to be responsible for something where the world looks full of hard decisions rather than easy ones?

I think some of this has just got to play out. What will help it play out is the broader public policy context and, if you like, the broader political context. I think the NHS has always seen itself as an island. It thinks it's different to every rule. For example, we have something called inflation, and we have health service inflation. We have employer/employee relationships in any other workplace, and then we have people called doctors. We have trade unions in other places, and then of course we have the BMA. Exceptionalism rules okay, in the NHS. That's been its characteristic.

But, actually, the context in which the NHS is now operating is changing. It is a world where it's all about devolution, it's all about localised control, it's all about getting difficult decisions out, it's about maintaining a more federalised system of governance in the United Kingdom in order to maintain the notion of the United Kingdom. The context for a secretary of state operating as the chief executive of a nationalised industry is being eroded every single day.

So, the self-same politicians who, when they get into Richmond House, decide that they're going to behave differently from how their colleagues, or even themselves, have behaved if they've had a different portfolio – I just don't think that's sustainable. It's the only one. It's the last man left standing. In every other arena – I mean Nicky Morgan [Secretary of State for Education] is no more in charge of schools than I am, is she?

So I think the ability to fight your own architecture just becomes more difficult, culturally.

So you ask does that mean that I think the idea of NHS England as a statutorily independent body is something that I broadly approve? Well, I think it is a stepping stone. I mean it's a monstrous bureaucracy. But it is definitely part of that.

Going back to my notion of an organogram, if I could choose to be the secretary of state that I wanted to be, I would like to be able to say, 'Hey guys, here's quite a lot of money. Here's a long-term plan with objectives against it. Not negotiated annually. But this is what you're going to get. This is the mandate. This is what you should go and do – though by the way I've got some real interest in helping to architect, not just the objectives, but the enablers.' The people at the top of any large organisation do not just sit there and think about strategy. They also think about the enablers to deliver strategy. So what's the workforce? What's the technology? What's the empowered patient? What is the stuff that you require in order to get you there? I'm not for a purist objective setting, strategy setting model, because I just don't think that in the end delivers the goods. It's not the real world.

In my experience this and every change happened through politics.

So in my experience this and every change happened through politics. Certainly in my time. Now I might have been either a terrible secretary of state, or I might have been just an aberration, but reform didn't come from the system.

Why do people, whether it's right or wrong, why do they now rather, through rose-tinted glasses, look back fondly on my time? Why? Because they feel that there was clarity. There was energy. There was determination. And there was shared mission because actually we were smart enough, I hope, to construct a shared view of what we wanted to do. It was because politics was driving it. So I think you've just got to be a bit careful with this debate because it can very easily turn into – 'if only the politicians got out of this, everything would be wonderful'.

If they do, fuck all would happen because what do systems do? What do bureaucracies do? They don't change. By definition they don't change so you've got to have a shock. Politics should be able to provide shock.

I think the thing that surprised people about when I was doing the job is how often I turned the heat on the NHS up rather than turning it down. If you're a Labour secretary of state, you're supposed to stroke it rather than kick it. I think you've just got to watch this a little bit… the 'if only we could depoliticise it, everything would be okay'. Equally, you've got to assure that the limits of politics are reached. I would say that the limits are around strategy, objective, and focus on putting the enablers in place that get the stuff delivered.

Take the Five Year Forward View. It is actually a menu of business models. That's what it is. It's not a strategy. Simon knows this. It provides a frame. But there's massive pieces of the jigsaw missing. What's the regulatory system? What's the workforce that will support this? What are the financial flows that will make it happen? How does it get implemented? All that sort of stuff is missing.

What Simon has done is two things. He has imposed a policy solution and he has imposed a resource solution on politics in a way that I've never seen happen. That is about his strength, absolutely. But it is also about political weakness. Burnham and Hunt have had to say, 'Yes, sir!' It's not supposed to be like that. Now, is it a good thing that that's happening, because it's Simon? Yes. Is it a sustainable or desirable model in a democratic system where there are accountabilities? Absolutely not.

Some of it needs to be about designing system architecture. And that should ultimately be for the politicians. Strategy and objectives alone are not enough. I don't buy the argument, to be honest, that the design of the system, the enablers that are going to make some objectives and strategy happen, are simply something that you simply absent yourself from. If that puts me in the Frank Dobson school of secretary of state-ship, which would be a very odd place to be, then in that sense it does.

If you want an exemplar of what happens when you remove politics from the National Health Service, I will cite in evidence Mr Andrew Lansley. What has happened? What has happened is that they've wasted five years; the system is in absolute turmoil. No one knows what they're doing. There is no clarity, there is no direction. Broadly, something that was broadly – broad brushstrokes – moving in the right direction is now broadly moving in the wrong direction. That's what you call the worst Secretary of State for Health ever and that's what happens when you remove politics. That's what happens when you put a policy wonk in charge of what inevitably has to be a system over which political judgements have got to be made. That's just how it is folks.

Let's take pay as an example: my biggest personal regret in my time. I think in terms of pecking order, I'd say the GP contract was actually pretty good because it basically tried to reward some of the right things. Agenda for Change – good in design, appalling in implementation. Consultant contract – a basket case. Now, if you go to the hospital in Valencia in Spain and you talk to the cardiologist, 40% of their pay every month is dependent on two things: the clinical outcomes they get and their patient experience scores. Their patient experience scores! 40%! And guess what? The quality of patient experience is pretty good and the outcomes are pretty high. Let's assume we wanted that and it was all left to Simon to design. Who do you think's going to have to answer for it when the BMA start marching on Richmond House? Or there's a lobby of parliament? Or the secretary of state is facing an opposition day debate because the doctors are going on strike? The idea that somehow or other the politicians will simply suffer the consequences and have no part in the design, seems to me at best to be naïve, and at worst fallacious. The politicians legitimately have a role, I think. That's why I said the enablers.

Do I want the Secretary of State for Health specifying how an A&E gets its waiting time down? Not really. Do I want the secretary of state to say this drug is better than that drug? Not really. Or nurse ratios? That's the responsibility of the people who are responsible for operating the system. The critique that one could make of this point of view is that it takes you back into Frank Dobson territory. But for me I'm very clear about where you go, and where you don't go. It's not to Cancer Drug Funds. It's not to earmark resources for x thing. It's not to specify how models actually work in practice. It's none of those things. But it does go beyond 'my job is purely to set the outcome, set the objective, set a budget and then hand it over'. Because, guess what, at best, I'm going to be responsible for the consequences.

My advice to a new secretary of state is really simple. Buy time.

My advice to a new secretary of state is really simple. Buy time. The best political trick I ever pulled off was to publish a 10-year plan. Why? Because it basically bought time. Because it said 'this is going to be a long journey, it's going to take a huge amount of time. I know that people are impatient for improvement and here's some milestones that I think we can achieve along the way'. But it's a 10-year journey, it's not a five-year one. I mean my experience in any walk of life is change always takes longer than people think – so buy time.

'The discovery of the overspend was a really shocking moment.'

Patricia Hewitt
May 2005 – June 2007

Rt Hon Patricia Hewitt was Secretary of State for Health from May 2005 to June 2007. She also held the posts of Secretary of State for Trade and Industry and Minister for Women.

Is the job impossible? No, it's not impossible, but it is unbelievably demanding. I think in some ways it's marginally easier for a current or new health secretary than it was when I took over in 2005, because what I found, very nearly 10 years ago, was a wholly inadequate leadership and capability within the department.

It was partly because the reform programme had been driven so hard by Tony Blair, Alan Milburn, then John Reid, John Hutton and the key special advisers. My impression when I arrived was that there were really almost no officials who actually understood what the reforms were about. So I think they had probably been somewhat disempowered, or had allowed themselves to be. It wasn't immediately apparent quite how deep the problems were. But it gradually became apparent.

The discovery of the overspend was a really shocking moment. As you know, the NHS is not allowed to overspend. In theory it cannot happen. But it did. The top of the department had absolutely no idea that there was a problem until three months into the new financial year. They finally got all the numbers and discovered they didn't sum to zero.

As we dug into what was really going on we discovered unbelievable inadequacies in the leadership, capability, and financial frameworks, and the discipline of the department and the NHS, in which the Treasury was also culpable.

When I say the officials – at this time the permanent secretary of the department and the chief executive of the NHS were one and the same person in Nigel Crisp. Richard Douglas, the finance director, who actually is very good, and is still there, wasn't even on the departmental board. A £100bn budget and the finance director isn't on the board! What world is this? He was buried below John Bacon, who was effectively, I suppose, chief operating officer.

So Nigel and the rest of them – about 13 of them – all came into my room and sat down along my very long table, with me, my special advisers and private secretary on the other side, and it was a complete 'Yes Minister' moment. It was the sort of, 'Minister, we have a problem'. And that was the overspend. That was a huge wake-up call and very nasty. It was later that I learnt from Ken Anderson, the commercial director, that there had been a series of pre-meetings about how they were going to gloss this problem to me!

The other very big wake-up moment was that I had been asking for a proper briefing on the reform programme – because I wanted to understand the new architecture that we were putting in place, and how we saw this 'quasi-market', the new system, working.

Nobody could give me a coherent explanation. Finally the permanent secretary said, 'Well, we've got a work programme for the reforms. Would you like to see that?' And I said, 'Yes, please!' And they came in with this enormous spreadsheet, which I always described subsequently as having 113½ different workstreams on it. The exact number was something ridiculous. I think it actually was over 100.

Anything that's got 100 workstreams for what is supposed to be a coherent reform programme, isn't coherent.

At which point I knew we had another massive problem. Because anything that's got 100 workstreams for what is supposed to be a coherent reform programme, isn't coherent. There was no change management strategy capability as far as I could see.

Then we had a crisis because the tariffs for that year turned out to be wrong. So we brought the tariff team up into the light and took a look at what was going on. And we discovered that basically we had three people – that's my recollection, it may have been four or five – struggling to create a tariff system. It wasn't their fault, but essentially they didn't have the expertise to do it. So we started sorting that one by getting people in from Victoria in Australia or the US and Germany where they knew how to do it.

And then there had been the decision by the officials – by the executive – to put out a document on primary care trusts that said – almost as an aside and without having run that part properly past ministers – that PCTs would be expected to get rid of their provider arms. That, of course, created appalling anxiety among district nurses and all the other tens of thousands of excellent staff affected. As soon as I realised, I withdrew the proposal and apologised. So it was just one thing after another. We didn't have the leadership capability or the structures that we needed.

Although the Lansley reforms have created the most appalling mess, and a lot of good people and capability have been weakened or destroyed in the process, there is also, I think, a very strong team in Simon Stevens and those around him. The independence, or greater degree of independence of NHS England, and the very clear responsibility that they have got for the NHS is, I think, helpful.

I was actually quite attracted by the idea of an NHS commissioning role. Later on I had very interesting discussions, both with my special advisers and with officials about it. And they just said, 'It's impossible. You cannot give away responsibility for £100bn. The secretary of state has to be responsible to parliament for that.' Now, actually the secretary of state remains accountable to parliament for it, even under the 2012 Act. But I felt very strongly that there were far too many issues, including clinical issues, coming onto my desk, in a very Nye Bevan way, really. The bedpan dropping in Tredegar.

It was quite ludicrous. And you needed a strong NHS leadership. At that point I was imagining you could have somebody like Ara Darzi* chairing the board, with a credibility in the NHS that no politician is ever going to have. That, it seemed to me, would make it far more possible to confront some very difficult issues, including reconfiguration.

Now, there's not much about the 2012 Act that one can admire. What Lansley did really was utter folly, in terms of this massive Act. This massive top-down reorganisation. The destruction of the PCTs and the SHAs, which then had to be recreated in different ways. All of that was unforgiveable, particularly at a time when those enormous increases in the NHS budget were ending. But the creation of the commissioning board – which in a sense was a logical next step from recreating the split between the permanent secretary and the NHS chief executive – I think that does have some merit. In any case, what you've got is a stronger leadership team – and with or without the commissioning board that's what you need as health secretary.

It was very odd coming from a much more classic Whitehall department [the Department of Trade and Industry] to move into the Department of Health, where most of the senior officials were NHS managers. There wasn't a strong Whitehall tradition there. But after Nigel went, with the help of Hugh

---

* Lord Darzi of Denham is professor of surgery and director of the Global Institute for Health at Imperial College, London. Between 2007 and 2009 he was the health minister in the House of Lords.

Taylor and Ian Carruthers, who were both brilliant, we gradually got to a much better place. And reintroducing the split between the permanent secretary and the chief executive was the right thing to do.

The distinction between policy and implementation is never as clear as people sometimes pretend. If you make policy without understanding both the constraint of implementation and the possibilities of implementation, particularly in the digital world, then you will get policy wrong. Therefore there is absolutely a risk, if you split in the way that the commissioning board does, then you weaken the input of implementation into policy. You have to guard against that.

The distinction between policy and implementation is never as clear as people sometimes pretend.

You've put to me, as an example, whether deciding to put extra money rather late in the day into winter pressures is policy or operations? Well I'm not close enough to it now really to be able to judge. But if the board [NHS England], and therefore the NHS management line if you like, say 'we are now at the point we're anticipating winter pressures, and factoring in the risk of worse flu than usual', something of that kind, 'we cannot any longer be confident that we're going to maintain the waiting times…'

They should then, in my view, come to the health secretary and say, 'This is the problem, and here are the options. We can relax the waiting time target – or rather you can. We can, if you give us additional resources, do this, that, and the other, and that will resolve the problem.' Maybe there are some other ideas. But, 'Here is the level of risk, and here are the options. It's up to you to decide which one you prefer. But if we don't get any of those then frankly we're going to have some pretty horrible headlines.'

You then have a sensible discussion. At the end of which the health secretary, and Number 10, and the prime minister, and the chancellor, decide what they want to do about it, and where they will take political pain, by taking money off other departments, finding it in the back pocket, or coping with the headlines or relaxing the waiting times, whatever it is. Now, to me that would be a grown-up conversation, and a sensible delineation of the respective roles.

What doesn't work is if you've got both NHS England and its board responsible for managing the NHS, and managing down the commissioning line – which was the mantra we kind of developed in my time, which presumably is still very much the mantra – but you've also got the health secretary, possibly with Number 10 and the chancellor as well, also wanting to micro-manage the NHS.

If you haven't sorted out the role of the health secretary, or you're not willing to sort out the role of the health secretary then of course it's not going to work. And you put it to me that we've both observed different health secretaries over the years and they behave very differently. That they want different levels of involvement in the detail and that trumps the formal arrangements. Well, yes. Of course! That's politics. And I do think from the NHS point of view that's pretty nightmarish, whatever the formal structures.

It would help if you had prime ministers who had thought more about health policy and the NHS

It would help if you had prime ministers who had thought more about health policy and the NHS, and how the two were best approached, before they became prime minister. And that then informed their choice of health secretary. The chance of that would be a fine thing! Not very likely to happen, but it would genuinely be helpful.

I'd observe that despite moving from one health secretary to another, there was quite a lot of continuity between Alan Milburn, John Reid and myself, because although we had somewhat different styles we were all basically Blairite reformers. Then the brakes got slammed on, really, with Alan Johnson and Andy Burnham.

That was partly because it had all got too difficult in my two years, and you needed to calm things down. I think you could have had one more year of really consolidating the reforms before you calmed it down in the pre-election period. I think under Gordon [Brown], Labour missed some opportunities there. And clearly, between Andrew Lansley and Jeremy Hunt, you have had a complete change of style, approach, and everything else! Wasn't he [Jeremy Hunt] at one point telling nurses to smile more? Honestly, it made you think he thought he was running a McDonald's franchise!

I do think the Five Year Forward View, which in a sense is NHS England's calling card to the new government – at certain levels there is quite a lot of continuity there.

If you look at what it says about not imposing another top-down restructuring, but not having 1,000 flowers blooming either, but really encouraging and getting behind developments that are already happening on the ground. That seems to me absolutely right, and very much where we had got to by 2007 – in terms, for example, of the relationship between the NHS and the local council, where there were joint budgets being developed, with joint commissioning and in a few areas there were joint chief executives between primary care trusts and local authority adult social services departments.

You had the beginnings of individual care budgets, and the possibility of extending those into health. A focus on how you integrated across organisation boundaries, around the individual. All of that. Which is what we were saying in *Our health, Our care, Our say*, which in many ways was the most exciting and constructive piece of work I did in my time as health secretary. It got rather overshadowed by all the crises. But Simon Stevens still refers to it. He absolutely sees the red thread remaining from that. Indeed, you could go back earlier to some of the fund-holding stuff and what Ken Clarke was doing. The line runs from that through *Our health, Our care, Our say* and on to today's Five Year Forward View. Now, okay it will take different organisational forms. And health secretaries will help or hinder, depending on what they're about. But underneath that, if you've got strong NHS leadership, centrally as well as in some localities, then a lot of good things are going to happen, even if more of them could have happened faster if Lansley hadn't thrown all the cards in the air.

Coming back to the questions about the board, if you've got one department which has got the NHS chief executive and the permanent secretary in it alongside the health secretary, you haven't got the sort of countervailing influence that an NHS England board can provide. I'm a great fan of Malcolm Grant [chairman of NHS England], and I think he's got some excellent people on that board. Potentially what that board gives you is an authoritative group of people, with a very deep understanding of the trade-offs and the pressures on the system, and that reinforces a strong chief executive and strong team around him. It has potentially got the advantages that you've currently got with monetary policy [the independent Bank of England] – although, of course, monetary policy is relatively simple in that it only has one objective while the NHS has many.

The Five Year Forward View is essentially a letter which says that 'with incredible effort on efficiency, and productivity gains, and some big changes in terms of behaviour, and prevention, etc we can close a large part of this gap. But we cannot close it all.'

I think that's really powerful. And it would be quite hard to do that with the chief executive within the department. Probably impossible. They could do it privately, to the health secretary. But that's a very different matter from doing it publicly with the authority of the board behind you. Of course there are disadvantages. But that strikes me as quite a big advantage, particularly in the highly uncertain political environment that the UK finds itself in.

You asked about inappropriate decisions that ended up on my desk. Let's start with reconfigurations. I felt we made enormous progress on that vexed question. When I came in John Reid had set up the Independent Reconfiguration Panel, but he hadn't used it, so we weren't sure how useful it would be.

The biggest reconfiguration problems started appearing on my desk, complete with attendant MPs, delegations, local publicity. One thing after another. But I sat down with the very good chairman of the Independent Reconfiguration Panel, Dr Peter Barrett, and got a sense of how he and the panel would approach things.

I spent a lot of time with MPs because the politics of these reconfigurations was a huge issue when you had MPs leading delegations, or going to Number 10, or leading marches. When that was happening, you clearly had a problem. These changes were all being damned on principle, because the public believed they were only driven by cost, and didn't regard that as a valid argument.

So we got the clinicians up front – starting with the clinical directors, the czars. We had George Alberti and Mike Richards and the others standing up and saying, 'If I have a heart attack or stroke, the last place I want to go is the local DGH [district general hospital]. Put me in an ambulance, or a helicopter if need be, and take me past whatever number of local DGHs, treating me on the way, and stabilising me, and get me to the hospital with the real expertise.' Once you get clinicians making that argument, it has a force that no health secretary can match. So that was a real breakthrough moment.

Once you get clinicians making that argument, it has a force that no health secretary can match.

We didn't succeed everywhere. But we were able with these wonderful clinical directors to overcome the wimpishness of some of the local clinicians who privately would say, 'Well, of course this maternity unit has to close', or 'actually, however reluctantly, yes, this children's heart hospital needs to close', or whatever, and would then publicly denounce the plans. And we got the NHS to get much better at consultation. And we then had the Independent Reconfiguration Panel which was good at picking up on very practical issues which the NHS was remarkably bad at in my day – for example that it was blindingly obvious that a maternity unit was unsafe but there was a huge issue around transport that needed to be addressed.

So we got many more of these reconfigurations through with that combination – much more clinical involvement, making the case, and with the Independent Reconfiguration Panel assessing the proposals and making recommendations to the secretary of state. I remember one Labour MP being absolutely up in arms about a reconfiguration, and I said 'why don't we refer it to the reconfiguration panel'? Some months later I asked what had happened, expecting mayhem to be breaking out around then, and was told it had all gone through. With some changes. But it had been approved by the local authority scrutiny committee and everything. So we did make some progress.

And then Andrew Lansley came along, after my time, and made this damn fool promise of an end to reconfigurations. He should have been shot. I was so angry with him. We'd managed to broker a way forward on Barnet and Chase Farm after something like 14 years and it all goes back up in the air. Richard Sykes and half the board of the London SHA resign. Years of hard work thrown away, although I gather now it has finally all gone through after some 17 years.

It doesn't always work. When I first became an MP in Leicester they were proposing to reconfigure three acute units into two and a half, so to speak, and it looked like it was going to go through until the politics stopped it. And blow me down, they've recently come up with another set of proposals to do roughly the same thing… After how many years!?

But by 2007 we'd got it to a place where you didn't have to have all those detailed conversations with the MPs. You would just reassure them that it would go to the independent panel, and they would consult. They would listen to the MP and everybody else and come up with a sensible solution, even when it was the same solution with a few tweaks. I thought I had really bequeathed a good, mature system for doing reconfiguration. Of the other things that came on to my desk when they should not really have needed to get there at all was the disaster around MTAS [Medical Training Application Service] and junior doctors' training. The new system had been designed reasonably well. But the execution was woeful. It was a shambles, a complete shambles.

I thought I had really bequeathed a good, mature system for doing reconfiguration.

You asked about other departments. I had been at DTI where I was also cabinet minister for women. There had always been deep tension between the Treasury and DTI. But I knew about the department, having been a junior minister for a couple of years. So I knew what was wrong with it. I just said from the outset, 'We are going to work seamlessly with the Treasury, as well as with Number 10. Special advisers will work with Number 10 and Number 11 special advisers. Officials, you are to talk to the Treasury. We are the supply side reform partners for the Treasury.'

I had that conversation with Gordon, and we led that from the top. Of course we still had some policy disagreement. But we could handle them sensibly. And with Geoffrey Norris as the special adviser at No 10, we just knew what we were doing. Every so often I would have a conversation with Tony [Blair] about something that was needed, or with Gordon. The one point where Gordon and Tony were on the phone several times a day was the Rover crisis during the 2005 election. But we knew it was coming. We had done a lot of scenario planning and built a team that could handle it.

When I moved to the Department of Health, I remember one of my special advisers who had moved with me coming into my office and saying: 'You've got to get Number 10 off our back.' They said DTI was fine, because we just talked to Geoffrey [Norris] once a week, and it was all very sensible. But my advisers at health were saying: 'Of course we know you're going to have regular meetings with Tony, and of course we know there's going to be a pre-meeting to prepare for the meeting with Tony. But when they're ringing us every day, and six times a day, and wanting to have a pre-meeting for the pre-meeting for the pre-meeting for the meeting, we can't get any work done. They've just got to give us enough space and enough trust so that we can actually do some work.'

We calmed all that down. There were a lot of changes on the health side at Number 10 as I arrived. Everyone was new, and that was another problem. Tony probably had the longest collective memory there! But after Paul Corrigan went to Number 10, and as I got to know David Bennett, who'd gone there as the head of the policy unit, the working relationships became very strong indeed. Both were excellent. And Tony had an instinctive understanding that the public wanted to be treated by the whole system as individuals who mattered, rather than being expected to fit in with whatever was most convenient for the system.

The policy was pretty well-developed. There had been all the targets, which had been Tony's preferred way of driving different behaviours to improve results across the public services, not just in health. On the one hand they were driving some really big improvements. But they did produce a culture where people were looking up, not out. And the way the financial performance was run from the centre when I arrived reinforced that.

You had the department telling the strategic health authorities and them telling the PCTs that: 'You've got to balance the books. We don't care how you do it, but you've got to balance them… there is only one correct answer, and that is zero in the right-hand corner.' So these magical cash-releasing efficiency gains would suddenly appear to give you exactly the right number to get to zero in the bottom right-hand corner – and they were fairy tales.

That culture of dictating from the top of the department, and not listening, meant the department probably genuinely didn't know – because it didn't want to know – that of course the NHS as a system, as a whole, was going to overspend. That was very shocking.

I ended up thinking that the intensely hierarchical nature of medicine, which on the one hand is necessary for clinical governance reasons, and patient safety reasons, but has been exacerbated over centuries by male consultants who are god, and female handmaidens who are the nurse, and all that highly gendered hierarchy in medicine, probably is particularly prone to a culture of bullying. The hierarchy slips into bullying.

I didn't think we understood that as a government. I've no doubt at all that the targetry, particularly on waiting times, compounded that command and control – the pre-existing command and control culture – and exacerbated the risk of bullying and harassment, and not listening to what was really going on.

I've no doubt at all that the targetry, particularly on waiting times, compounded that command and control

So we were trying to get to a 'self-improving' organisation, in the phrase that Matthew Swindells, my special adviser, and I came up with. One that would 'look out, not up'. So choice and competition, and foundation trusts and the tariff as ways of encouraging local innovation, and in my last few months, introducing NHS Choices and extending choice. We were trying to embed those reforms so that they would become irreversible. Though choice and competition were expunged from the vocabulary the minute Tony and I left!

My advice to an incoming health secretary? Be very careful. What may appear to be quite a limited change in structures, or in the law, may turn out to be like pulling on a piece of thread and unravelling everything. The reorganisation I did in 2005, which was driven by a commitment to release efficiency savings – we genuinely wanted and believed it could be a bottom-up reorganisation. But I then started discovering that the department was just basically ringing around the NHS and saying, 'Oh, never mind what she said. This is the answer. This is what the reorganisation is going to be in your area.' They didn't begin to get the idea of bottom-up. Back to the command and control structure. So we had to get rather involved in that as well! I do think you have to be very careful, and do a great deal of listening, in order to understand as far as possible what the unintended consequences might be of apparently well-meant changes.

'Piss off. I'm dealing with this.'

Alan Johnson
June 2007 – June 2009

Rt Hon Alan Johnson was Secretary of State for Health between June 2007 and June 2009. He was also Home Secretary and Secretary of State for Work and Pensions, Trade and Industry, and Education and Skills.

I don't think when a bedpan falls on the floor in Tredegar it should echo around Whitehall anymore. I think that kind of command and control model was very much a creature of its time. With the population queueing up, grateful for what they'd got, deferential to the clinicians, so you had a service that was basically built around the convenience of the clinicians.

A consultant would book everyone in at 9:00. They'd all be there, and he wouldn't waste a minute of his precious time waiting for someone to arrive. Parents weren't allowed to go and visit their children. There were 150 hospitals that didn't allow any visiting at all to children. And the rest? I remember going to see my sister when she was in for appendicitis. You could only go for an hour on a Sunday afternoon. It was almost charitable.

When I was as the department you wanted the service to be clinically led, locally driven, but you wanted a secretary of state who was the accountable face of it, the only accountable face of it, and to be able to pull a lever and something happened.

I was very much in favour of the first line of the Act [Health and Social Care Act 2012] – that the secretary of state would be responsible and accountable, which Lansley tried to change and was pushed back on. I saw that as very important. There was absolutely no way that I would have set up this huge quango, NHS England, to protect ministers from that. There was no way I would have pursued that because it was never going to work. Parliamentarians aren't going to put up with being told, 'Nothing to do with us. Write to NHS England.'

Now I mean when Mid Stafford broke, Bill Moyes [the Chairman and Chief Executive of Monitor] was trying to tell me that was his responsibility and not mine [to remove the chair and chief executive of Mid Staffordshire NHS Foundation Trust] – because it was a foundation trust. Now politically it would be very nice if you could get away with it and say, 'That's yours. That's your can of worms.' But I told him, you know, 'Piss off. I'm dealing with this.'

Now David Nicholson saw this danger very early on about the way Monitor, especially under Bill, was very serious about taking total control and being in a way separate from the NHS. Even if Moyes had been able to cope with the public scrutiny it just wouldn't be fair to the public or to him for that matter. You're the secretary of state. There is public money going in there. You are responsible. We had plans to row that in [the independence of Monitor] if we'd got back after 2010. But it was Stafford in particular that made you see the consequences [of the idea of an independent board].

You're the secretary of state. There is public money going in there. You are responsible.

Bill was probably right that the legislation said he was responsible. So you are probably right when you say that if you feel yourself, as the secretary of state, to be accountable, the legislation may say this, but… In a place like health [you are accountable], anyway, because it's very different to the DWP

[Department for Work and Pensions] and the Home Office and education. You try to do that with the police, or the head of MI5, it would be a ludicrous thing to do.

But in health you are making the administrative decisions. Do you close that hospital? Do you move that chief executive? Those administrative decisions have to be with the secretary of state because they impact.

On reconfiguration I stepped out of the firing line. I announced two things on my first day. No more top-down reorganisation because the NHS was sick of it, and that was important because the Darzi Review could have been seen like that, when really it was genuine bottom-up. But the other thing I said was 'I'm making no decisions on reconfiguration'. The Independent Reconfiguration Panel had been set up by John Reid. They were clinically led – good people on there – and they made their report, and referred it for the secretary of state's decision. I made it clear I'd back them. I said, just so that I didn't entirely tie my hands, I said, 'I can foresee no circumstances in which I would intervene.' They make the decision.

Andrew Lansley very stupidly tried to reopen all that. But take Manchester. For 40 years they were trying to configure maternity services in the Manchester area, and it was costing babies' lives. Everyone knew that. The Manchester local paper was brave enough to support it, but everyone was defending bricks and mortar. That was why it hadn't happened. But in the end they got what they wanted, a much better, much safer maternity service. It wasn't for me to say that the clinicians were wrong on that. You want the service clinically led.

You asked me about choice and competition. I could see the argument for moving away from that dreadful kind of 1948 'you put up with what you get'. I could see that. There were millions of people using the health service, and basically they were treated very badly under the old system. That needed to change. So if you called that choice and competition, fine, but it never really got my juices flowing.

But I did set up the Co-operation and Competition Panel which was there to rule on the application of competition law in an advisory capacity. I can't remember much about it. It did its stuff and I don't remember it ever causing us any problems, which is a measure of its success. And now Andrew Lansley has turned it into this monster through legislation, so now we have competition lawyers sitting in the corner every time two hospitals talk to each other.

If we get back in, we have to get rid of all that competition stuff in the Act, so we get rid of the lawyers and find a way that helps people integrate their services. But it will be important that people don't perceive this as another top-down reorganisation. So NHS England has to stay. Simon Stevens is well known to us, and I am sure we'll find a way to make that work.

I say the secretary of state was responsible, but actually it was a quartet. I've never known any other department like it. So there was me, but there were three permanent secretaries of equal status – the permanent secretary, the chief executive of the NHS and the chief medical officer. The CMO has been downgraded a bit, and unfortunately, because Sally [Davies, the current CMO] is brilliant.

I've never known any other department like it.

We had plans to downgrade the CMO as well if we'd won the election. Liam Donaldson was a great guy. But he wouldn't share his annual report. He would just publish it, and he wouldn't give you any knowledge of what was in it or anything. Well that's not a triumvirate working together. That's one separate empire. So that had to be reined in a bit.

And there were things I didn't want to do that Gordon insisted we did, like free prescriptions for patients with cancer. Every time a conference came around, Gordon wanted something to say on health. But all prime ministers do that. They want to say something on health – so what can you fish up? It can be eye-rollingly difficult.

Health is different to the other departments. You've got that triumvirate for a start. You've got a much bigger budget. You've got the daily grind of issues that come up to a much greater extent than anywhere else – because, you know, Mrs Jones fell out of bed in a Portsmouth Hospital and was seriously injured, and they want to be seen in their local paper to be raising it on the floor of the House. And you get a whole series of adjournment debates [on particular issues] which thankfully I [as the secretary of state rather than the minister] didn't have to deal with. But you knew you were more in the public eye, and you had this vast empire. How many people? 1.3 million! Like the Indian railways etc. And you don't directly control them. But for the public, they kind of think you do. They think you've got control. I had a woman come to my surgery asking me to write to the Secretary of State for Health on an issue, and I was the Secretary of State for Health… I said, 'That will be no problem. I'll get that done for you!' I think that is totally inescapable in a tax-funded health system, but it is a small price to pay.

And in my time health was a bit different because you could throw money at a problem. The same was true to an extent at education, and even a bit at DWP although I was only in DWP for seven months, but that was less true at the Home Office.

My advice for an incoming Secretary of State for Health? Make no major speeches for at least a month. Find out exactly what's going on there. Decide what you want to do in that time because you'll get a honeymoon period. People won't expect you to be doing very much.

Wherever you can, defer to clinicians. If there's an issue there, and clinicians take one view, and politicians take another, go with the clinicians, on reconfigurations and the big clinical issues. And that's partly because, unlike any other department, when the staff aren't happy then you're an unpopular secretary of state. It hurts in health. It doesn't really hurt in the Home Office, or even in education. Because if teachers are unhappy with you, it doesn't mean to say that parents are – in fact quite the opposite sometimes.

In health, if doctors and clinicians don't like you, you can be absolutely sure that all their patients won't. It feeds through very quickly. Of course you will have your battles with clinicians, over GP opening hours, say, or with overblown consultants. But at least make sure they're the right battles.

'It's a hard balance. It's very hard.'

Andy Burnham
June 2009 – May 2010

Rt Hon Andy Burnham was Minister of State for Health from May 2006 to June 2007 and Secretary of State for Health from June 2009 to May 2010. He was also Secretary of State for Culture, Media and Sport and Chief Secretary to the Treasury.

The job as I see it is to get the best possible health care – the safest, highest quality health care – for the people of England. And to protect them from health risks. I guess that's it really.

On the question of scope, and the separation between management and policy, we did look at having an independent board. I think this went back to about 2005. Will Hutton, the journalist, wrote a book called the *The State We're In*[*] and that proposed a constitution for the NHS and the separation of management and policy. It was around that call that you hear that 'we need more stability, less politics in the NHS'. I looked at the idea of a board quite seriously. I thought the constitution idea was valuable, because it would make everybody clear about their rights and responsibilities, and politicians' rights and responsibilities. I thought that had value.

---
[*] Hutton W. *The State We're In: Why Britain is in crisis and how to overcome it.* Cape, 1995.

The board was discussed at the point of transition [between Tony Blair and Gordon Brown] and Gordon's team got interested in it. But when we thought about it, it quickly dropped away when you thought about the implications. So we backed off.

You simply cannot have £100bn-worth of public money without democratic accountability. I remember people saying you couldn't have MPs writing and the secretary of state saying 'oh, don't ask me', which is kind of what happens now.

You simply cannot have £100bn-worth of public money without democratic accountability.

If politics has a respectable role, it's obviously in providing accountability for taxation. And if that doesn't apply in respect of the NHS, then what does it apply to? We backed off. I think the foundation trust reform in many ways was our answer to it. So more autonomy at a local level, but you still need that national accountability.

What's going on at the moment doesn't really work. And I think this government has realised it doesn't work. There are a number of things I could say. For example, Jeremy Hunt has a Monday morning meeting with all the organisations. He's been ringing up hospital chief executives, which if I did that it would have been a very rare thing to do. I can't recall doing it.

Where organisations had got into difficulty was different. I recall speaking to the chief exec of Basildon I think. Obviously when I inherited the immediate aftershock of Mid Staffs, I appointed the chief executive there. To be honest I inherited a very difficult situation, which actually took me away from the idea of independence because when I arrived in the department in 2009, the trust at that point had an interim chief exec and an interim chair. And I said, 'Hang on a second, this is after a terrible meltdown here, why haven't we got the best in the NHS in that hospital now?'

The answer was, 'Oh well, [it is] Monitor – they don't want to put anybody in. And you set up Monitor and it's your foundation trust reform.' I basically at that point realised that it just doesn't work in that scenario. You have to be able to override systems, and the requirements for public safety and good governance means that politicians will occasionally have to step in.

So yes, occasionally I had contact with them [chief executives], but not in the way Jeremy Hunt does, definitely not. I'm told he picks up the phone all the time. It's completely counter to the reforms they've put through. He has a Monday morning meeting, I'm told, with Monitor and CQC and others. Now we hear they've got a cabinet subcommittee that is monitoring NHS performance and is issuing quite stern edicts to the system, almost daily, saying, 'We've noticed your delayed discharges are a bit off target, get them sorted out and reply to us by tomorrow.'

I think they've realised it just doesn't work in practice.

I'd like to pull it back in some way, restore the secretary of state's duty, with respect to providing a comprehensive health service. It doesn't mean that you then pull everything back in. The chief executive, who was based in the department, probably could sit outside of the department and that is a healthy thing – that arm's-length arrangement. It's not about saying we just get rid of NHS England. There is a respectable case to be made for running the NHS separate from the government structure, outside the department. There is a debate to be had about statutory independence. But that would imply that they could ignore or refuse to do something, as Monitor did refusing to replace the chief exec at Mid Staffs so we forced the issue just because it wasn't acceptable to me.

Alan Johnson had to face the same issue [in dealing with Monitor over Mid Staffordshire]. He had put the interim chief exec in place on the back of that and then that was it. That was as far as they [Monitor] were going to go.

I think this government has found that when well-meaning reforms collide with reality it's the test of whether they are the right reforms. And they've often been found to be wanting. I'd even say this government has been operating in a more top-down fashion at times.

But I do think it's good if secretaries of state don't get too involved. It's a hard balance. It's very hard. This is why I would stand by the foundation trust reform, not exactly as it was conceived, because we're going to have to update it. But the idea that there is more autonomy at local level, in terms of operations and how visions and things should be implemented. That's a good thing. That is where a good level of independence is needed at local level. Getting the balance right does then become a question of personality. It becomes an issue of people's style, and do they carry people with them, and how do they go about their job?

There are clearly different styles for doing the job. It all depends on the context, it really does.

There are clearly different styles for doing the job. It all depends on the context, it really does. I would encourage you to think about this, because every secretary of state operates in a different context. I'll give you two things I know very, very well. Number one was a financial meltdown, which you remember well, in 2006/07. It's one of those things where the system almost collectively loses its way. It does need to be one by one brought back into a proper financial position. And I would say something similar is happening now, where financial discipline has broken down to some degree and it probably needs something similar. I saw Patricia do that, and it was successful.

The second example I'll give from my time, which was swine flu. That goes back to my very first comment about responsibility to protect the public, arguably that's the primary duty, before you get good health care for everybody. The pandemic was declared three days after I arrived in the department – so talk about Teflon Johnson, the man with the best timing in the business!

People think about Mid Staffs. But the thing that was most immediate for me was swine flu. I remember being in the secretary of state's office, asking, 'What does it mean?' They explained the arrangements that were going to kick in – 'Gold Command' and all this kind of thing. I remember David Nick [Nicholson] winking to me saying, 'We're in command and control mode now.' It was a self-reflective, self-deprecating, joke. But it was important. We did have to go into that mode, very much so. And people wanted us to. Very clear advice, instructions to PCTs, instructions through NHS Direct. We did have to have some negotiations with the GPs. But once that had been done, it had to be implemented in full. In those early days when the pandemic had been declared, it was pretty serious really.

When the Lansley reforms came along, we said, 'What are you going to do in a similar situation?' The beauty of the secretary of state's power is that it's there. Yes, in ordinary times you would expect an individual to use it with a very light touch and permissive feel. That would be the ideal. But there will be moments where, because it's there, you can use it to its full benefit to protect the public. That is what we did and although swine flu wasn't as bad as people feared, it was frightening for a while.

And then there was the NHS constitution. As Patricia Hewitt's deputy, I was tasked by Tony Blair to really think through the next stage of reform, and how do we move a bit beyond the turbulence that had come from the financial depression. I picked up this sense, when I'd gone out and about doing work shadowing, that NHS values were being frayed and a bit of up for grabs and 'where is your reform going?' I proposed the NHS constitution as a way of anchoring the service again. Bringing it back together a bit. Refocusing it. Putting some things beyond doubt that needed to be put beyond doubt. I put it together, but it was really Will Hutton's idea.

Between that time from being minister to secretary of state [for health], I was Chief Secretary to the Treasury and then Secretary of State for Culture, Media and Sport. There is a big contrast between those jobs and health.

All departments have a very different feel, they really, really do. The feel of the Treasury is, 'We don't have to listen to anybody. This is where it's at. Who are these people out there?' That's the feeling there. The feeling in DCMS [Department of Culture, Media and Sport] is, 'Why would we try and do anything? We're so weedy.' And then DH [Department of Health] is more self-confident than that, but…

They all have their own culture informed by the service beneath them. I was in the Home Office for a little while – so I went Home Office, DH, Treasury, DCMS, DH. The Home Office definitely has a very tough, no-nonsense feel to it – because of the police involvement and prison involvement. But I like DH. I think I warmed to it more. Friendly but very worldly wise.

Health is probably more political as well. Not necessarily party political. But in terms of the people believing in the thing that they're in. I don't think you get that in other government departments in quite the same way – both a professional vocation but also an emotional belief and connection to what they're doing. Public health is always I think quite radical, and quite outspoken, for good reasons. There's a bit of idealism there that definitely you don't get in Treasury or Department for Culture, Media and Sport. Or even the Home Office, where you're responsible for a whole load of things that you can't do a great deal about. So yes, it does have a very different feel to it.

In terms of advice to an incoming health secretary, there are a couple of points. It's so much more about the people on the ground than people ever realise – the sense of their engagement and understanding of what you're trying to do. I think Whitehall sucks you in, to the department and all these national bodies. I think Jeremy Hunt understands this better than others who have done the job, to be fair to him. And having a plan for the workforce should be the first thing that you do. Really getting that sorted out, making sure that morale isn't going to dip, and you've got a grip of training and enough numbers coming through. Just having a people strategy, honestly. It's almost the last thing they want to talk to you about in the department, but that feels to me to be the first thing really.

I did that quite a bit through what we called the Social Partnership Forum with the employers, but mainly because we had let our eye off that ball a bit, and we needed to get back on it. I think this current government has suffered for the lack of a good workforce strategy, under the Lansley reorganisation. As that was going on, they were making frontline staff redundant and now they're stuck post-Francis with this agency bill.

And it gets more important in financially strained times rather than less important. You might think, 'God, anything to do with the workforce will cost money.' But it costs money to neglect it – you get the agency bill growing, overseas recruitment, all this stuff. It really pays dividends to get a proper grip on that. So that's number one.

You might think, 'God, anything to do with the workforce will cost money.' But it costs money to neglect it

The second thing I would say is I think the position is more parlous than people realise, in terms of where the system is right now. I would say if people are embracing the notion of integration in their different ways and from their different vantage points, it's something that needs to be embraced wholeheartedly, in all of its implications. By that I mean I would take a moment to reset expectations about the NHS. The journey ahead of it. How services are going to have to change. How people might have to take responsibility for their own health a bit more. How it can't be used like a consumer service because it's not a consumer service. It's a customer service based on 'you take what you need, but you take no more than what you need'.

I think it needs to be re-explained to people in that context and expectations reset. So that the NHS has some breathing space to start to make some changes they probably should have made many years ago, around switches from the hospital to home and integration. I look back at Patricia Hewitt's white paper and it was way ahead of its time – *Our health, Our care, Our say*.

That's the issue now. It's the only show in town as far as I can see. You really have to get the public to understand that process, and buy into it, and establish some degree of consent for that to happen. Those are the things. I mean there are the immediate firefighting issues that have got to be done and quickly. Some financial discipline has to be restored. The thing you hear in the NHS all the time at the moment is, 'We can please CQC or we can please Monitor, we can't please both of them.' You have to quickly sort that out. But in terms of the two big priorities, I would focus on those two.

'The more you try to do,
the more you get hit for it.'

Andrew Lansley
May 2010 – September 2012

Rt Hon Andrew Lansley was Secretary of State for Health from May 2010 to September 2012. Later he was Leader of the House of Commons.

The secretary of state should be the representative of the public in the stewardship of the National Health Service, and on behalf of the government to take responsibility within government for the public health.

I was particularly conscious of the imbalance that my predecessors struck in being overwhelmingly concerned with the internal behaviour of the NHS, while acting in essentially a responsive manner in relation to public health.

So my view was that in order for the NHS to function more effectively it required long-term stability, and – it will not surprise you to know – short-term change in order to bring long-term stability. A sense in which the secretary of state – while responsible with the government for the provision of resources and the legislative framework, and for the stewardship overall of the system – would not be interfering day by day in decisions which should probably be made by the NHS.

That in itself would allow the secretary of state to take a far more proactive position on public health. Which is why I wanted to publish as rapidly as possible a public health white paper – about how the government understand and have an impact on the behavioural change we are looking for. A structure through which we could work with the public, local authorities, charities and the private sector in order to try and deliver some of the changes in risk factors which would be essential to improving public health. I know you want to hear about the NHS. But I think it's quite important, because in truth, in two and a half years through the establishment of Public Health England, the structure of the white paper – some of the measures we took through the responsibility deal and the further tobacco control measures – I actually think in terms of progress in a couple of years on public health we did more than, I could honestly I think say, any of my predecessors in a comparable period of time. Even stretching back all the way to Ken Clarke. Many of those risk factors, underlying risk factors were moving inexorably in the wrong direction with a few honourable exceptions. Pretty much, we are starting to see corners turning on some of these public health measures.

You put it to me that I wanted there to be a Secretary of State for Health – a proper Secretary of State for Health – and merely a minister of state who would worry about the NHS bit. I know. I did ask them that. And David [Cameron] said, 'All right, later. Once you've done all the legislation.' When I'd done all the legislation I moved on, so he didn't feel obliged to do it.

Now, the NHS relationship. From my point of view, and we've had this argument and you know my point of view, the idea that you could just do this stuff without legislation – well it's for the birds. The whole point was that I knew perfectly well from recent and painful experience of my predecessors that trying to do NHS legislation is a nightmare. I therefore resolved to do it once and hope my successors would hardly ever have to do it again. Because the institutional structures in the NHS would be proofed for the longer term.

We will only know in 10 years' time. I think it would be an enormous blessing to my successors if they did not have to legislate again. I'm always amused by Alan Milburn's detailed critique of what I did wrong. I got my legislation. He didn't get his, not in the form he wanted it. I did get it, and I got it in the form which if you've talked to the secretaries of state back to Ken Clarke you will know that, as Stephen Dorrell has said, with the exception of Frank Dobson, every secretary of state basically wanted a structure like that. They wanted to deliver, after 20 years, a purchaser/provider split that was real. They wanted to strengthen commissioning, but often found they were in a provider-dominated system. They wanted to create a system which was focused on the interests of the patient rather than the interests of the provider.

I think it would be an enormous blessing to my successors if they did not have to legislate again.

I believe the system is consistent with that, and it has created a voice for the NHS. In my view the Five Year Forward View published last October is compelling evidence for the benefit of the 2012 Act. Because it set up NHS England – gave NHS England that voice. Of course health is a vitriolic debate in the election. But it isn't fundamentally about the view of what the NHS should be doing over the next five years – because that's set out in the Forward View and nobody's argued with it. All the political parties are pretty much subscribing.

So they're trying to have a vitriolic debate about narrower and narrower issues, like do you give them £2.5bn more than they have asked for, or do you give them £3bn more than they've asked for? In particular where the issue of integration of health and social care is concerned, it's pretty much a completely trumped-up debate – because the integration of health and social care will happen. The structure is there through the health and wellbeing boards which it wasn't before. Local authorities are engaged in health to a degree they never were before. GPs, through clinical commissioning groups, as commissioners, have a vested interest in designing systems which support their activity in the community in looking after patients in a way that never happened. PCTs never did. They were obsessed with the target culture and that was hospital driven not community driven.

There is serious money in the Better Care Fund – for good or ill. Also personal budgets, which if you actually want to integrate health and social care in practice is, in my view, the only way you can really achieve it – enabling people with chronic conditions to combine health and social care. Otherwise, I don't know what integration looks like frankly, because in the absence of that you have top-down institutional silos that still argue with each other. Or you end up, like Alan Milburn did, announcing children's trusts on the basis that because there is one children's trust everything relating to children will automatically be integrated. Five or six years later you realise it hadn't happened at all because actually all the professional silos were continuous.

I have worked in other departments and was a full civil servant. And the fact of the matter is that, if you are Secretary of State for Health, the more you try to do, the more you get hit for it. The secretaries of state who the NHS probably likes best are the ones whose obsession is with doing nothing. Frank Dobson basically just wanted everything to go back to how it was. Which was – I don't mean to be unkind – populist but purposeless. Patricia Hewitt tried to do something to be fair to her. She would probably tell you – probably has told you – I gave her hell for it, because she was trying to do things. Alan Milburn tried to do things and in truth

The fact of the matter is that, if you are Secretary of State for Health, the more you try to do, the more you get hit for it.

his political career stopped at that point, though by his own decision to some extent.

Alan Johnson didn't try to do anything really. He just tried to respond to a few things that turned up. Andy Burnham there was no time. And he was obsessed with social care anyway. He did try to do something with social care which time doesn't permit me to explain the vacuity of the white paper that he published on social care before the election, which Labour now will pretend was some answer. It was no answer at all.

So do I think the idea of creating NHS England as a separate commissioning board to take politicians out of the day-to-day decisions on the NHS has been a success?

I think it is a work in progress. I think it is evidently a success to some extent. For example, take the Cancer Drugs Fund. We are where we are partly because politicians, my successors, collectively failed to see through the policy, which was to move to a value-based pricing system by 2014. Living with the consequences of that is NHS England, which is sitting down with NICE, with the Medicines and Healthcare products Regulatory Agency and the charities and patient groups, and they are trying to work this system out now. They're not depending upon ministers to do it. So that's evidence of progress. The Five Year Forward View is evidence of progress.

You note I said 'work in progress'. And you put it to me that some people would say that the contrast between I and Jeremy Hunt couldn't be larger in that I absolutely believe in the split which I legislated for, and that he's been petty and interventionist on a whole bunch of things.

Yes. He's trying not to be, but he gets draw in, and of course that will be true for all secretaries of state. The law is what the law is and there are limitations. And let's face it, on the mandate, behind the scenes Malcolm Grant and Simon Stevens last year took the opportunity to say, 'No. Thus far, but we're not doing all these things that you're asking for, we'll negotiate.' The NHS in the past never had any negotiation, never had a voice, so it is an effective internal voice as well as an external voice. In a way the NHS Executive never was.

It never was, though it was intended to be. That's why I don't think what I was trying to do was novel in that sense. That's what Ken was trying to do with the NHS Executive. Which is why in cabinet Ken Clarke sat there and basically every time we discussed this said, 'I agree with all of this.'

You put it to me that in practice the behaviour of different secretaries of state, and they all behave differently, will always trump the legislation. Yes. You could argue that. And the response to Mid Staffs is suggestive of that. Because the NHS, left to itself, would never have introduced specific nursing to patient ratios across hospitals.

The NHS will develop over time an underlying sense of their own statutory wellbeing. You can see it; it will take time. Clinical commissioning groups are starting off employing people from former primary care trusts, some of whom sit around waiting for NHS England to tell them what to do, even though they have the power do it themselves now. Other people are coming in and saying: 'We've got a budget and the power now. We can do stuff. We should.' Of course there's a whole load of accountability structures. But actually if they do stuff, with the health and wellbeing board and the local authority working with them, for NHS England it's actually quite hard to stand against it when it comes down to configuring services and making decisions.

The NHS will develop over time an underlying sense of their own statutory wellbeing.

At the end of the day you have to say, 'Did it work?' The long run – in so far as it was designed to create long-running stability for the NHS in terms of structures and powers – we will only know in 10 years' time.

In the short run, I have to say, 'What were we trying to do?' We were trying to maintain the outcomes and improve them with a budget that was only going to go up by 2–2.5% cash a year. Whereas they'd got used to 7– 8% cash a year. This was very different.

We are now four-and-a-half to five years down the line. I haven't gone through the most recent data. But I think if you did you would find, pretty much, the outcomes are at least as good. There's no fundamental difference. People talk about accident and emergency waiting times. That's not an outcome. That's a process measure. If you actually look at the outcomes, I think we're doing at least as well. We're doing it with more clinical staff despite the constraints, and we're doing it with 21,000 fewer administrators.

You asked about the job relative to other secretaries of state. I think only the Ministry of Defence has a comparable situation where a large body of the people who work inside the department, to the secretary of state and ministers, operate to their own agenda if you like. A professional agenda – calling it professional dignifies it – but an agenda of their own, which is not the one that ministers have necessarily given them. That was certainly true in the department. That was principally managers in health, but also doctors who had gone into the system and just liked it. The whole structure of clinical directors – the czars – had ballooned. Nobody in the department had any idea why we had so many clinical directors.

There were czars for everything, and they didn't want anything to change. They liked being czars, but it was a fundamentally unaccountable position in many ways. They just got to kind of pontificate on everything.

You've asked about how far you can divide policy from management or operations. But you're assuming I was dividing policy in the department from operations in NHS England; I wasn't. I was working on the basis that the Department of Health would set the statutory framework and would only intervene in policy at the highest level through the mandate. So if it's not in the mandate they [the department] shouldn't be [intervening], no. I think they're still intervening – of course they are – but it will get harder and harder over time.

To which you say but Jeremy Hunt has set out policy on hospital food and car parking charges, or whether you put an extra £200m into winter. He knows he shouldn't. But I think sometimes, when you look at it, it's stuff which NHS England has in practice decided and ministers are badging for political reasons. As time goes on, after the election Simon [Stevens] and Malcolm [Grant] and Bruce [Keogh], they should take ownership. Last year for example, the whole 24/7 agenda – providing a proper seven-day service because too many people are dying at the weekends – ministers deliberately didn't take it over. It could have been a ministerial agenda; in the past it would have been. Ministers would have fronted it. But no. Bruce is fronting it and that's actually going better. Still BMA are against it because BMA are against everything. But it's much more likely to succeed because NHS England is leading it.

You put it to me that the white paper said NHS England would be 'a lean and expert organisation'. And it became somewhat larger than that.

Well, it is not simply a headquarters. It actually does do the commissioning of primary care and the commissioning of specialist centres, the commissioning of dentistry, optical services and pharmacy. There's a load of operational people as well as the people who do the policy and the headquarters stuff. As long as we've got the administration headcount down and costs down by a third and we keep it moving downwards – which is actually NHS England's intention going through; if I'm correct there's a current process for a further round of rationalisations – then we're moving in the right direction.

You will have seen the National Audit Office [July 2013 report] which concluded on the transition that it had been done on time and on budget, and concluded that it was an immense achievement.

The NHS departmental accounts last year show, if I remember correctly, a gross cost of the reforms at £1.4bn and a net benefit over the parliament of between £5bn and £5.5bn, and a recurring £1.5bn a year reduction in the administration costs of the NHS. So the idea that it created some kind of bloated structure is nonsense.

That it created a structure that people don't understand – absolutely, but then nobody has ever understood the way the NHS works. People who worked in the NHS, in my repeated experience, had no idea what the structure for decision making in the NHS was. If you said to them, 'There's a thing called the NHS Executive,' they'd go, 'Is there really? I thought it was in the Department of Health.' You'd say, 'Yes it is in the Department of Health.' They'd say, 'Well, it's the Department of Health then isn't it?'

People who worked in the NHS, in my repeated experience, had no idea what the structure for decision making in the NHS was.

Classically we had this ridiculous situation where people were very unhappy about the closure of a ward in their local hospital. So they all went to the primary care trust to complain. The primary care trust said, 'It's nothing to do with us, it's all been decided by the strategic health authority.' So they went to the strategic health authority who said, 'No, it's nothing to do with us it's to do with local decisions by the primary care trust.' So they went to ministers. And the minister says, 'We're not responsible for it, it's all being done locally.'

Alan Johnson was very keen on all these decisions being made locally by the primary care trust. He was rabbiting that one out all the time when I was on the other side of the despatch box. I was ranting at him saying, 'You keep trying to claim credit for everything that goes right in the health service, but you try to say every local primary care trust is responsible for everything that people don't like. Nothing to do with you.'

To him Maidstone was nothing to do with him. Mid Staffs was nothing to do with him. Morecambe Bay. None of it was anything to do with him. It was all to do with the ghastly people out there.

So you put it to me that first Alan Johnson would not describe it that way and second that I tried to create a system that made that true. I did. Because it is true. But he pretended otherwise. He tried to control everything and take credit for everything and then pretend that it was all local. Well, it is now, because the law sets it out. Statute sets out who is responsible, and actually the difference within Mid Staffs is that the commissioners barely touched the surface of the problem.

You put it to me that NHS England are statutorily responsible for the delivery of A&E waiting time targets and all the pressure they are under this winter. But there is a big political row about it. Well, there always will be, I can't take that away. I didn't actually, to be fair to you, make it clear – I couldn't take the politics out of the NHS. I could to some extent take the politicians out of it. Then, of course, what you have is politicians arguing with the same noise level about a restricted number of things. And that is in fact what they're doing. They are actually arguing about one or two targets, and money, and not much else actually because there isn't much else to argue about.

…I couldn't take the politics out of the NHS. I could to some extent take the politicians out of it.

It may work. I don't think it's naïve, but I think it is optimistic to see this particular change happen quickly. If you go to other countries, you very largely see politicians out of that debate. They do get drawn back in occasionally like in France… Bertrand who is the French health minister and for some reason I was talking to him in a hospital in Villeneuve or somewhere, and he said, 'The number of times I've had to get involved in that one.' So they do get involved, but much less.

So it is not removing politicians. It is at least restricting them. Trying to hamstring the politicians a bit. Of course, we will only know in 10 years' time if it's worked – if there are not annual reorganisations of the NHS. I did have to have what was undoubtedly the biggest reorganisation it has seen. But in order not to have every new secretary of state walk in the door and issue a new white paper that changes all the structures. That is what happened, because they could. Because the law pretty much said the NHS is whatever the secretary of state of the day at any given moment decides it is. Now we actually have a proper statutory definition of what it is, how it's run, who's in charge of what – it is all there.

You put it to me that it is possible it won't get changed for many years not so much because it is all working perfectly but because the row that was generated by what I did means that no one will want to do it again. Yes, that is entirely possible, and that is also deliberate.

They'll live with whatever they've got, because nobody in their right mind will try to argue with it. If there were a Labour government in three months' time, in my view there will not be a repeal [of the 2012 Act]. What they will try to repeal is Section 75. Officials will explain to them carefully that by taking the competition powers for Monitor out of the health legislation, they will simply give all the same powers – exactly the same powers – to the Competition and Markets Authority who will exercise them in a far more aggressive way, if they choose to do so, than Monitor. So they'll blanch slightly at that thought and walk away from it.

As for the remainder, Labour agree we should have NHS England. They agree we should have clinical commissioning groups. They agree we should have Healthwatch. They agree we should have health and wellbeing boards. They agree we should have Public Health England. That's all settled.

Two more things I need to mention. One social care: we didn't do Dilnot how we should have done it, because we are now having to put a shedload of NHS money into backing up the social care activity. The level at which the cap on care costs is set is still too high. We will not get the market to respond at this level.

I was very clear on what we should have done. We should have funded Dilnot by removing the exemption for the property that a person lives in from the domiciliary means test. I pushed for that. And the Treasury wouldn't have it. The reason they wouldn't is because there are 200,000 people at any given time who are in receipt of domiciliary care – and whose means test is to that extent very generous to them because their property is not taken into account.

Amongst that 200,000 would be 100,000 who benefit from a Dilnot-type system with a lower cap because an extra £1.5bn or so would be going into supporting people who reached the cap. The way the numbers worked we would have been able to say nobody would ever have to commit more than 40% of their assets to meet their care costs. Whatever level of assets in the UK, never more than 40% of their assets.

But the Treasury kept saying that 200,000 people would lose and 100,000 would benefit, so we are not going to do it. So in the end the Treasury was willing to actually find their own money, but less of it, to do a high cap. The cap should have been at £35,000 not £75,000 because then the insurance market might work. However, we did put in the structure. So it only now requires extra money to get to the point where we can unlock Dilnot's system.

My advice to an incoming secretary of state? Firstly, keep being the patients' voice. Work with Healthwatch and the patient groups to get that, so that when the public hear you speak they hear a genuine reflection of their own view of the NHS. Secondly, recognise that it's your job to ask for improving outcomes. It's not your job to tell doctors and nurses how to do it. Thirdly, if you really want to make the biggest difference for the people we represent, focus on how we deliver better public health. Everybody actually knows that making the population healthy is not delivered through the NHS, it is delivered through almost everything else, so just focus on all that stuff. Be the voice for public health inside government. Which is very difficult at the moment because when I left David Cameron shut down the cabinet subcommittee on public health.

Part 3:

*The views of the former
Secretaries of State for Health on…*

…restricting the role of politicians

William Waldegrave 'Is it possible, in any business or in any organisation, truly to separate policy from execution? I certainly thought then that to see the policy through, I had to retain the strategic control of what was happening with some kind of non-party political support. You shouldn't be, as the secretary of state, accountable at all for the providers, except that, for reasons of history, the great majority of the providers, belonged to the state. So, you had to be at least accountable for them not stealing the money, and audit and propriety and so on. The theory was that the minister should do the prioritising, but not run the services.'

Alan Milburn 'I think you've just got to be a bit careful with this debate because it can very easily turn into – "if only the politicians got out of this, everything would be wonderful". If they do, fuck all would happen because what do systems do? What do bureaucracies do? They don't change. By definition they don't change so you've got to have a shock. Politics should be able to provide shock. I would say that the limits are around strategy, objective, and focus on putting the enablers in place that get the stuff delivered.'

Stephen Dorrell 'But all this stuff about creating independent decision making and getting the health service out of politics blah, blah, blah… Well, that's exactly the same speech that we used to make in favour of the health authorities that were statutorily independent. They existed in statute. They had responsibilities defined in statute. So what's changed?'

Andrew Lansley 'I couldn't take the politics out of the NHS. I could to some extent take the politicians out of it. Then, of course, what you have is politicians arguing with the same noise level about a restricted number of things. And that is in fact what they're doing. They are actually arguing about one or two targets, and money, and not much else actually because there isn't much else to argue about. It may work. I don't think it's naïve, but I think it is optimistic to see this particular change happen quickly. So it is not removing politicians. It is at least restricting them. Trying to hamstring the politicians a bit.'

Andy Burnham 'You simply cannot have £100bn-worth of public money without democratic accountability. If politics has a respectable role, it's obviously in providing accountability for taxation. And if that doesn't apply in respect of the NHS, then what does it apply to? I'd like to pull it back in some way, restore the secretary of state's duty, with respect to providing a comprehensive health service. It doesn't mean that you then pull everything back in. But I do think it's good if secretaries of state don't get too involved. It's a hard balance. It's very hard.'

Frank Dobson 'You put it to me that my period was seen as a period of strong command and control because there were a lot of centrally decided initiatives – setting up NICE, and the Commission for Health Improvement, National Service Frameworks. Well, I entirely agree with that. I have no problems with command and control. It is part of the secretary of state's job. As for the current split of NHS England as a statutorily independent commissioning board? Well it is bollocks. The idea that the NHS is going to be this independent organisation, without political interference, and this, that and the other, is just rubbish and it has proved to be just rubbish.'

Virginia Bottomly 'How far can you take the politics out? Well Ken [Clarke] set up the NHS Executive in Leeds to try to get that sort of separation. That involved an awful lot of first class tickets, and chat on trains! Ken absolutely believed in principle that the executive and the trusts should be more autonomous. He absolutely believed that politicians should be away from the direct management. My instincts were more to worry away, if there was a problem, know what the problem was. The old bedpan metaphor continues to run.'

Kenneth Clarke 'Every secretary of state has been trying to de-politicise the daily management of the system, detach themselves from it, because the political arguments are ludicrously unhelpful. But faced with huge petitions and MPs lobbying you in the House of Commons you will never entirely get away with saying "This is nothing to do with me. I have no powers over this." I think we're a long way from ever achieving that. But we'll see how it goes. The reason I think it is working so far is that the board [NHS England] is not actually asserting itself as a rival centre of power. It is actually giving a clinician-led – apparently clinician-led – lead to policy making.'

…the Lansley reforms

Andrew Lansley 'Of course, we will only know in 10 years' time if it's worked – if there are not annual reorganisations of the NHS. I did have to have what was undoubtedly the biggest reorganisation it has seen. But in order not to have every new secretary of state walk in the door and issue a new white paper that changes all the structures. That is what happened, because they could. Because the law pretty much said the NHS is whatever the secretary of state of the day at any given moment decides it is. Now we actually have a proper statutory definition of what it is, how it's run, who's in charge of what – it is all there. In my view the Five Year Forward View published last October is compelling evidence for the benefit of the 2012 Act. Because it set up NHS England – gave NHS England that voice. You put it to me that it is possible it won't get changed for many years not so much because it is all working perfectly but because the row that was generated by what you did means that no one will want to do it again. Yes, that is entirely possible, and that is also deliberate. They'll live with whatever they've got, because nobody in their right mind will try to argue with it.'

Alan Johnson 'There was absolutely no way that I would have set up this huge quango, NHS England, to protect ministers from [public accountability]. If we get back in, we have to get rid of all that competition stuff in the act, so we get rid of the lawyers and find a way that helps people integrate their services. But it will be important that people don't perceive this as another top-down reorganisation. So NHS England has to stay.'

Kenneth Clarke 'I'm the only politician in the House of Commons who says that Andrew Lansley's reforms, on the whole, seem to be quite beneficial, and once they settle down they'll have a good effect. The scale of disruption in introducing them was ridiculous. That enormous bill was just hubris. I argued to him that he didn't need a bill. That that all of it, certainly almost all of it, could have been done within his existing powers. The reason Andrew failed was because he couldn't explain it. He got immersed in all the technicalities and, even I couldn't follow what he was going on about. He needed some broad brush stuff, instead of which he immersed himself in the detail so that nobody understood it, and everybody got fearful that some dreadful change was being made. It was over-elaborated. But the underlying point was OK. So I supported Andrew Lansley's reforms.'

Alan Milburn 'What has happened is that they've wasted five years, the system is in absolute turmoil. No one knows what they're doing. There is no clarity, there is no direction.

Broadly, something that was broadly, broad brushstrokes, moving in the right direction is now broadly moving in the wrong direction. That's what you call the worst Secretary of State for Health ever and that's what happens when you remove politics. That's what happens when you put a policy wonk in charge of what inevitably has to be a system over which political judgements have got to be made. That's just how it is folks.'

Patricia Hewitt 'Now, there's not much about the 2012 Act that one can admire. What Lansley did really was utter folly, in terms of this massive Act. But the creation of the commissioning board – which in a sense was a logical next step from recreating the split between the permanent secretary and the NHS chief executive – I think that does have some merit. Although the Lansley reforms have created the most appalling mess, and a lot of good people and capability have been weakened or destroyed in the process, there is also, I think, a very strong team in Simon Stevens and those around him. The independence, or greater degree of independence of NHS England, and the very clear responsibility that they have got for the NHS is, I think, helpful.'

Stephen Dorrell 'I voted for the 2012 Act and there were reasons why I did so, and I am quite happy to defend why I voted for it. You've heard me say it, times without number, that actually health policy hasn't changed. Frank Dobson would like to have changed it and wasn't able to. But apart from him, no health secretary has wanted to change policy since 1991, which is the day when it really did change. We used to have a provider-led system; we now have a commissioner-led system. That is different, but it's the last time anybody fundamentally changed health policy.'

…the Department of Health

Andy Burnham 'All departments have a very different feel, they really, really do. The feel of the Treasury is "We don't have to listen to anybody. This is where it's at. Who are these people out there?". The feeling in DCMS is, "Why would we try and do anything? We're so weedy." And then DH is more self confident than that, but… They all have their own culture informed by the service beneath them. The Home Office definitely has a very tough, no nonsense feel to it – because of the police involvement and prison involvement. But I like DH. I think I warmed to it more. Friendly but very worldly wise. Health is probably more political as well. Not necessarily party political. But in terms of the people believing in the thing that they're in.'

Patricia Hewitt 'Is the job impossible? No, it's not impossible, but it is unbelievably demanding. It was very odd coming from a much more classic Whitehall department [the Department of Trade and Industry] to move into the Department of Health, where most of the senior officials were NHS managers. There wasn't a strong Whitehall tradition there.'

Kenneth Clarke 'I always joke with Jeremy [Hunt] that being minister of health is a political deathbed in most western democracies. In every western democracy, health is the most controversial subject that politicians encounter, because it's so emotional and there are such tensions and competing interests. It's also one of the most important.'

William Waldegrave 'Secretary of State for Health is the most powerful managerial job in Whitehall, or was then. If you were a powerful enough minister with enough coherence and enough support from senior management, you could actually change things. Even the Secretary of State for Defence can't do that. The Chiefs of Staff can just say, "No," and go to the Prime Minister if they want to. The job at Work and Pensions, [where there are tens of thousands of staff delivering benefits] might be comparable, but I never did that one.'

Alan Johnson 'Health is different to the other departments. You've got a much bigger budget. You've got the daily grind of issues that come up to a much greater extent than anywhere else – because, you know, Mrs Jones fell out of bed in a Portsmouth Hospital and was seriously injured, and they want to be seen in their local paper to be raising it on the floor of the House. In health you are making the administrative decisions. Do you close that hospital? Do you move that chief executive? Those administrative decisions have to be with the Secretary of State because they impact. It's very different to the DWP and the Home Office and Education. You try to do that with the police, or the head of MI5, it would be a ludicrous thing to do.'

…key moments and turning points

William Waldegrave 'When I was appointed, Mrs T [Thatcher] said to me, "Kenneth [Clarke] has stirred them all up, I want you to calm them all down again," and then made it absolutely clear to me that if I wanted to just cut the throat of all these reforms that was fine as far as she was concerned. I then went along with Duncan Nichol and we had a meeting with her in Number Ten, just before she went to Paris, just before she fell. We persuaded her, and it was a matter of persuasion, that the thing made sense and wasn't just Kenneth trying to cause trouble.'

Alan Johnson 'When Mid-Stafford broke, Bill Moyes [the chairman and chief executive of Monitor] was trying to tell me that was his responsibility and not mine [to remove the chair and chief executive] – because it was a foundation trust. Now politically it would be very nice if you could get away with it and say, "That's yours. That's your can of worms." But I told him, you know, "Piss off. I'm dealing with this."'

Andrew Lansley 'The idea that you could just do this stuff without legislation – well it's for the birds. The whole point was that I knew perfectly well from recent and painful experience of my predecessors, that trying to do NHS legislation is a nightmare. I therefore resolved to do it once and hope my successors would hardly ever have to do it again. Because the institutional structures in the NHS would be proofed for the longer term. We will only know in 10 years' time. I think it would be an enormous blessing to my successors if they did not have to legislate again.'

Andy Burnham 'People think about Mid Staffs. But the thing that was most immediate for me was swine flu. I remember being in the Secretary of State's office, asking "What does it mean?" They explained the arrangements that were going to kick in – "Gold Command" and all this kind of thing. I remember David Nick [Nicholson] winking to me saying, "We're in command and control mode now." It was a self-reflective joke. But it was important. We did have to go into that mode, very much so. And people wanted us to.'

Patricia Hewitt 'The discovery of the overspend was a really shocking moment. As you know, the NHS is not allowed to overspend. In theory it cannot happen. But it did. The top of the department had absolutely no idea that there was a problem until three months into the new financial year. They finally got all the numbers and discovered they didn't sum to zero. As we dug into what was really going on we discovered unbelievable inadequacies in the leadership, capability, and financial frameworks, and the discipline of the department and the NHS, in which the Treasury was also culpable.'

…style and behaviour

Alan Miburn 'Why do people, whether it's right or wrong, why do they now rather, through rose tinted glasses, look back fondly on my time? Why? Because they feel that there was clarity. There was energy. There was determination. And there was shared mission because actually we were smart enough, I hope, to construct a shared view of what we wanted to do. It was because politics was driving it.'

Kenneth Clarke 'It wasn't command and control, although there was this mad illusion that I was supposed to command and control it. That I was sitting there in the middle with all these thousands of staff. I think I was the first to point out that it was the largest employer in Europe apart from the Red Army. You were of course held responsible every time anybody dropped a bedpan, and somehow you had a huge administrative structure, which ensured that you controlled all this. It was hopeless. It was a gruesome, self-perpetuating bureaucracy, riddled with vested interested. It was collapsing.'

Stephen Dorrell 'I did try to behave like chairman of the board, not chief executive of the National Health Service. But when people said to me what did I think about the coalition setting up an independent board, I used to say "well I am the person who abolished the last one!"'

William Waldegrave 'I made myself the chairman of [the policy board]. It was implicitly saying that the secretary of state should not just be policy, but should also be an executive. Perhaps I shouldn't have chaired it. But then this is the inherent difficulty of the whole thing – is it possible, in any business or in any organisation, truly to separate policy from execution?'

Andy Burnham 'There are clearly different styles for doing the job. It all depends on the context, it really does. I would encourage you to think about this, because every Secretary of State operates in a different context.'

Virginia Bottomley 'The one thing [Margaret Thatcher] said, which always stuck in my mind, is "never turn down the opportunity to explain the government's case, because nobody else will". The other thing I felt, this is an organisation that's got a million people, there are patients, users who are all very emotional and "No comment" isn't good enough. The message needs to be communicated.'

Frank Dobson 'I believe Simon Stevens once referred to me as wandering up and down the ministerial corridor in my stocking-ed feet, like the non-executive chairman who knew what he was doing. I took that as a compliment really.'

…advice for the next incumbent

Alan Johnson 'Make no major speeches for at least a month. Find out exactly what's going on there. Decide what you want to do in that time because you'll get a honeymoon period. People won't expect you to be doing very much. Wherever you can, defer to clinicians. If there's an issue there, and clinicians take one view, and politicians take another, go with the clinicians.'

Kenneth Clarke 'Know what you are doing, get stuck in and enjoy it. Health secretary was probably my biggest single challenge. The two jobs I've enjoyed most were Health and the Treasury. I'm not sure which I enjoyed most, the Treasury probably, because you get into every form of government. But I enjoyed health. It was the toughest job I ever had, much tougher than the others.'

Frank Dobson 'I was much criticised because I said to some reporter from the *Daily Mirror* who came to see me that the first thing I was going to do was sit down and have a good think! Which is out of fashion really isn't it, to sit down and have a good think? I think they need to do that.'

Andy Burnham 'It's so much more about the people on the ground than people ever realise. I think Whitehall sucks you into the bodies and the Monitor and the this and the that and actually having a plan for workforce should be the first thing that you do.'

Patricia Hewitt 'Be very careful. What may appear to be quite a limited change in structures, or in the law, may turn out to be like pulling on a piece of thread and unravelling everything. I do think you have to be very careful, and do a great deal of listening, in order to understand as far as possible what the unintended consequences might be of apparently well-meant changes.'

Stephen Dorrell 'Stick to the policy that all health secretaries except Frank have pursued – of developing commissioning. In the end, the health secretary is the commissioner in chief. So actually, they should stop obsessing about hospital management, which is anyway a fraction of care delivery. Recognise you're commissioner in chief, accept responsibility for the commissioning process, and make it work.'

Alan Milburn 'Buy time. The best political trick I ever pulled off was to publish a 10 year plan. Why? Because it basically bought time. Because it said 'this is going to be a long journey, it's going to take a huge amount of time.'

About the authors

Nicholas Timmins

Nicholas Timmins is a senior fellow at the Institute for Government and the King's Fund. Between 1996 and 2011 he was public policy editor of the *Financial Times*. He is also a visiting professor in social policy at the London School of Economics, and at King's College, London in public management. He is a senior associate of the Nuffield Trust.

Edward Davies

Edward Davies joined the Health Foundation in September 2014 as a Policy Fellow. Edward has spent the majority of his career working as a health journalist. Most recently, this saw him working as a North American Editor for the *BMJ* and, prior to that, writing for a range of trade and general publications from *Medeconomics* to *the Guardian*.